THE FOOD ADDICT:
Recovering from Binge Eating Disorder & Making Peace
with Food

Additional books by Merry Brown
The Four Families Series
Gold Manor Ghost House
Crimson Hall Ghost House
Silver Tree Ghost House
Serpent Star Ghost House (spring 2022)

The Exiled Trilogy
The Knowers
The Second Fall
The United

YA Books imprint
ISBN 978-0-9899934-5-6
September 2021

All web links and addresses were valid at the time this book was published. Due to the changing nature of the internet, some links may no longer work.

Front and back cover designed by Merry Brown.
Front cover photography, Alicia Field Pinto.

Forward

The roots of this book go back to the summer of 2009. I'd
had an epiphany and wanted to share what I'd learned with
the world. I wrote a diet book about making peace with food
through the use of the virtues, chief among them self-control. I
was convinced the only way to battle food addiction was to
fight, each and every day, against my inordinate desire for
food. Bootstraps dieting.

By the end of 2009, I lost the rigid control I'd tried to exert
over my eating and fell headlong into a binge eating disorder
and depression. By the summer of 2011, I was able to go off
anti-depressants and I embraced my new way of life: no diets
ever.

Since I was done with dieting, I assumed the diet book I
wrote would forever be buried in my computer, never to see
the light of day. I certainly didn't want anyone to read it.

Getting over my embarrassment, I have married the old and
new me in this book. I took excerpts, when possible, from the
old book and amended them. I've also included lots of
glimpses of what it looks like to live in a mind that has a food
addiction. A decade ago, I couldn't see the sickness for what it
really was. I knew I was sick, but the remedy I offered was
toxic: the sickness was eating too much, the remedy was self-
control.

I no longer see the sickness and cure this way. My malady is
a physical and psychological disorder, and as such, the cure is
found in medical and psychological treatment.

My great hope for this book is to offer solidarity for those
who suffer from food addiction and to offer insight for those
who don't. Since no two people are the same, the suffering
differs as well. This is my story and long road to recovery.
While your story is different, I hope you will see you are not

alone. There is hope for you to end your suffering and make peace with food.

Table of Contents

Introduction

I've been overweight since my freshman year of high school, though my disordered eating began long before it showed on my body. While body size doesn't tell you if a person has a food addiction or disorder, our culture likes to pick on and discriminate against fat people. We like a good fat joke.[1]

The easy explanation for (and subsequent solution to) obesity is to place blame on the fat person.

Problem: you (fat person) eat too much.

Solution: stop overeating through self-control.

Problem solved, right?

This is the solution, the easy answer, to the obesity epidemic. But is it really? Tell me, who is this easy for? It has the obese on a constant diet struggle, the odds never in their favor. The mental health, physical health, and financial weight is carried by our entire society with this false narrative.

So, I ask again, telling overweight people to simply eat less (problem solved), who is this easy for?

This false and shallow understanding of body size is "easy" and advantageous for:

- The 72-billion-dollar diet industry[2]

---

[1] Two things as we begin. First, not all people who are overweight have a food addiction. Food addiction has nothing to do with the size of the body. Food addiction is a mental health issue. Secondly, this book is about my experience in the world. I've been overweight since I hit puberty and have therefore experienced the world from that perspective. I am aware that people who are below the normal weight range are routinely picked on too. Our culture will bully anyone for just about any reason. But, given my experience, this book only examines what it's like to be overweight in a thin-obsessed culture.

[2] https://www.businesswire.com/news/home/20190225005455/en/The-72-Billion-Weight-Loss-Diet-Control-Market-in-the-United-States-2019-

- Vast segments of the 2.5 **trillion**-dollar global fashion[3] and 532-billion-dollar beauty industries[4]
- People who want an easy way to feel better about themselves while (culpably) misunderstanding others

This book examines and exposes the lie that the whole story about our complicated relationship with food rises and falls with self-control.

People are over and underweight for a whole host of reasons. You cannot tell what is going on with someone by looking at them. We do not assess someone's health from a visual glance.

For those who suffer from disordered eating, I want you to consider this: your illness is along the same lines as the cancer patient or the clinically depressed. Something is wrong.[5]

Blame is irrelevant and counterproductive. Do we waste time shaming and blaming the person whose clinical depression is due in part to poor choices? Do we tell that person to just get "over it?" We (should) know better. The depressed person has a condition that needs to be treated. Let's treat the entire person.

Do we waste time blaming the person with cancer because he lived in an area with known carcinogens? Do we say, "You

---

2023---Why-Meal-Replacements-are-Still-Booming-but-Not-OTC-Diet-Pills---ResearchAndMarkets.com

[3] https://markets.businessinsider.com/news/stocks/the-richest-fashion-designers-and-brand-moguls-in-the-world-2017-9

[4] https://www.businessinsider.com/beauty-multibillion-industry-trends-future-2019-7

[5] I am addressing, specifically, people who suffer from disordered eating. I am NOT talking about people who are overweight. There are different eating disorders, and within each eating disorder, millions of individual ways in which they are lived and experienced. I don't want to make the mistake of asserting that everyone with an eating disorder, or specifically BED, thinks and experiences the world as I do.

should have moved. Your cancer is your own fault?" We (should) know better. People who live around known environmental hazards stay for a variety of reasons. How the person got cancer is not the focus. The person now needs medical treatment.

What about food disorders? I'm not concerned with causation, the past. I'm concerned with the present. What can I do now? If I'm trapped in a pit, why spend precious time poring over how I got there? The prudent action is to recognize the condition, "Hey, I'm in a pit! I don't want to be in a pit. I want out. Help!"

How do you get out of a pit? It depends on you and the pit. Is there a rope? Do you have the ability to climb it? How deep is the pit? Are there other people in the pit you can help and can help you? Are there stairs in the pit? Maybe even an elevator?

When I was trapped in binge eating disorder, I was alone in a mile deep five-foot-wide black hole. I was there with my incessant thoughts. It was awful and debilitating.

I found my way out of the deep misery of binge eating disorder. It is my hope as you read about my experiences you will know you are not alone and you, too, can find your way out of the pit of despair to the fresh air of freedom. Away from binge eating disorder and towards a life of making peace with food, your body, and your mind.

SECTION I: MY LIFE WITH FOOD

Chapter 1: The Early Years

When did I become overweight? Puberty. I was not an overweight child and did not have a weight complex in grade school. Nonetheless, even as a child I coveted sweets. I stole cookies from the cookie jar, I made bike runs to the 7-11 mini mart to get candy bars, four for a dollar. One of my favorite treats at the 7-11 was a tub of chocolate frosting. Yum! I would take it home and hide it in my room. It would last me at least two days.

As a child I was a hider. I hid what I was eating so no one would, what? Judge me? Make fun of me? No. So no one would say "no" and take my sweets away. Sweets. I love sugar and sugar loves me.

On to the mid-1980s and puberty. Around the beginning of 8th grade, I started filling out. By the time I got to high school I was overweight, not obese, but enough to feel unlovable, to feel less important than others who had no extra weight.

My high school was great for those who loved useless sugary foods. There was a snack shop at my very large school that had all manner of junk food delight. My usual lunch, before I had a car and drove off campus for fast food, was a bag of sour cream and onion potato chips, candy bar or hostess treat, and a coke.

To make matters worse for my hips and heavenly for my tongue, I worked in a yogurt shop throughout high school. Now, taken in moderation, frozen yogurt is not that bad for you. I, however, am not a moderate eater.

I lacked self-control when it came to all things food. The chief reasons I would stop eating were: First, the treat was gone and I had no money or opportunity to buy more. Secondly, I felt like I was being watched and stopped because I didn't want to be labeled a pig. Finally, because I could not physically eat anymore, which was usually why I wasn't eating at any given time.

Working at the yogurt shop I had access to all kinds of treats. We had every kind of topping I desired from Butterfinger bars to peanut butter cups to hot fudge to sprinkles, and, of course, plenty of frozen yogurt. We also made waffle cones that were dipped in chocolate and smothered in a variety of candy or nuts.

I ate my way through high school. I did my stint with bulimia. I threw up because I didn't want the calories, only the taste. But, since I'm trying to be honest, I usually threw up so I could eat more.

In high school I tried a variety of diets. I tried Jenny Craig, counting fat, not eating, throwing up, counting calories, etc. My favorite diet was the one that started in the morning. Tomorrow morning, that is. That must mean I should treat myself to a big farewell dinner, dessert, and maybe one more dessert since it's going to be my last - for a while.

I was mostly resigned, already, to this being my life. The happy fat girl. The good friend.

When I got to college in the fall of 1990, I weighed somewhere in the 170s at 5'1". I had an excellent college experience. My freshman year, I lived in a dorm on campus and had a meal card. Most of my friends complained about the cafeteria food, and I did too – just to fit in. In truth, I was delighted! You mean I could eat anything I wanted?!? I could go back for as many treats as I desired or could psychologically stand people seeing me eat? Oh, the cafeteria – the land of milk, honey, and unlimited cereal.

Many of the friends I made that first year in college suffered the traditional fate of the first-year college student known as the freshmen 15 – the amount of weight loads of students pack on their freshman year of college. I gained weight too, but didn't notice much. Several of my friends worked on their bodies over the summer, returning to school in the fall with relatively the same shape they had when they began school the previous year. I didn't even consider seriously dieting that summer.

I loved college. I learned a lot, had tons of fun, and adored my friends. I didn't date in college, not because I wasn't willing, but because no one was willing to date me. This was painful, but not unexpected. I hadn't dated in high school either. I attended proms and formals but only because in each case I asked the guy. Geez, this is a hard thing to remember.

It's not that I thought I was repulsive; I was likeable and fun to be with. I never blamed the males for not picking me, given all my pretty friends. My friends were date worthy; whereas, I was friend material. I wanted to date so badly. I was sure the lack of male attention was due to my weight and yet I felt trapped in my body. I felt powerless to change my eating habits, and honestly, didn't want to eat like a bird.

I obviously had self-esteem issues. I suppose I was comparing myself to the women on the cover of *Cosmo* or *Seventeen Magazine*. The movie star, she was desirable. She had the body men wanted. Who would want mine when something better could be found? It turns out the women on magazines had been photo-shopped and air brushed. Regardless, there were better bodies around me, and my body tempted no one.

In hindsight, my body issues were ridiculous. I was smart and fun; could I help it if the male population around me were idiots? Nonetheless, I think a huge part of my problem was my own embarrassment. I was so embarrassed by my body, so uncomfortable in my own skin, I unconsciously invited others to view me the way I felt I deserved.

My only semi-successful college diet came the spring semester of my senior year. I was about to graduate and move across the country to Kentucky for graduate school. This was an exciting and uncertain time in my life. I adored my undergraduate college experience and was sad it was coming to an end. I wanted to get control of at least one aspect of my life since I didn't have any idea what the future held. I ate a low calorie, low fat diet and began walking.

By the time I moved to Kentucky in the fall of 1994, I had lost about 20 pounds, down to my lowest weight in memory at about 158 pounds, and I was sick of dieting. I was still going through the motions, but my heart wasn't in it anymore. I was tired of eating crappy food and denying my appetites.

I did one of those weird diet moves and lied to myself, saying, since I had lost weight, it was okay for me to eat more. And boy did I!

I met my husband-to-be two weeks after moving to Bowling Green, Kentucky. He was also a new graduate student in the same program. We hit it off right away and were married within a year.

Christopher loves to eat good food. Even in the beginning of our relationship he would cook for me. He was thin his entire life and used to having a high metabolism. He could eat a tub of Ben and Jerry's and not gain an ounce.

Once he graduated from college his metabolism slowed and he began to put on weight. He hadn't changed his eating habits, but his body had changed. By the time I met him in graduate school he was about 20 pounds overweight.

As the years stretched on, we grew together, literally. My love for him grows and deepens every year. Unfortunately, my dress size was going up and up too, along with his expanding waistline.

When we completed graduate school, we moved to St. Louis in the fall of 1997 for Christopher to work on a Ph.D. in philosophy at St. Louis University. It was in St. Louis that I joined Weight Watchers for the first time. My weight was back in the high 170s.

I really liked the Weight Watchers program. Counting points was easy for me. I stayed on the program for about three months, following my usual diet pattern, and lost about 20 pounds again. I felt great *and* deprived all at once.

How could I spend so much time and mental energy losing weight and still gain it back? It's not that I don't know what causes me to gain weight. So why in the world would I commit so much time, money, and energy to something just to throw it all away?

Very perplexing. It's hard to explain to the person who doesn't have weight issues why most of us don't lose weight and keep if off. It is so irrational to gain what one fought so hard to lose. Needless to say, I gained the weight back, *plus* an additional 20 pounds.

Five years into our marriage I became pregnant with our first child. I now weighed 195 pounds. I knew typical women without food issues can easily gain 30 pounds plus while pregnant. What was going to happen to me?

One of my St. Louis friends became pregnant around the same time I did. She was about 6 weeks ahead of me in her pregnancy. Laura was tall, thin, and beautiful. She was a truly radiant pregnant woman. I watched as she grew and how her body changed. I wanted so much for others to see that I was pregnant too. I knew people attributed her growing belly to pregnancy and mine to being fat.

It's not that I looked hideous pregnant. I often joked that I looked better with a pregnant belly, for it helped to balance out all the weight in my butt, thighs, and hips. I just wanted others to see my pregnancy and smile, like I imagined they did when they looked at Laura.

Luckily, I didn't gain much weight, only about 10 pounds total. I'm not sure how I escaped gaining 30 pounds or more. In fact, in the first months of pregnancy I lost a bit of weight. It wasn't due to being nauseated, because being sick to my stomach rarely kept me from food. My eating didn't alter much during pregnancy. I was used to indulging my cravings anyway, so satisfying my pregnancy induced cravings didn't feel that new to my body.

Soon after the birth of my first child in the summer of 2001, I was back in my regular clothes. The ten pounds I'd gained was mostly baby weight plus fluids.

When our son was nine months old, my husband and I went on Weight Watchers together. I joined the program again and I gave him the information. *This was the first diet my husband had ever been on!*

In the span of four months, he lost 50 pounds, going from being in the 230s to the 180s! Let me tell you this now if you do not already know: it is entirely unfair to lose weight with a man. He lost between two and four pounds every week to my one and half-pound losses.

In addition to his mega weight loss abilities, my husband does not have "food issues" beyond liking food a lot. He responded quite differently to his change in diet. He did not appear to be desperate, unduly deprived, or obsessed with the when, where, and how much of dieting. In fact, from the very beginning he saw himself as not being on a diet as much as having changed his lifestyle. How did he get to be so psychologically healthy?

What did my husband do to lose the weight? He cut out sugar soda and went to diet soft drinks, he paid attention to his portions, limited dessert to one time per day, and exercised about three days a week. The weight melted off. He was overweight because he had not made the adjustment from his boyhood days to his new adult body. I suspect my husband has never felt the need to hide one piece of food he has eaten.

On this diet with my husband, I lost about 30 pounds, going from around 195 to 165. Towards the end of this diet, we moved to a small town in Tennessee. I went from working full time to being a stay-at-home mom in a town where I knew no one. And, oh yeah, living out in the country. We only had one car at the time and my husband used it to get to work.

The weight came back.

I went on another diet in the fall of 2004, the year after my second son was born. I tried Weight Watchers again, this time without formally signing up and going to meetings. I lost about 40 pounds and was *convinced* this time I would keep it off. I had a yard sale in early summer and sold all my fat clothes. By summer's end I was kicking myself because I didn't have anything to wear!

The weight was back.

Chapter 2: My Last Diet Ever

The beginning of my Last Diet Ever happened on June 4, 2008, the day I took my mother to the airport. She was visiting from California for a few weeks, and we had a wonderful time together.

While she was here, it struck me that she looked better than I did! I always *knew* my mother looked better than me because she weighed a whole lot less and looked good in her clothes, whereas I was heavy, unhealthy, and my clothes were too tight. Well, it hit me, just hit me, that I did not look good *and* my mother looked better *and* she was 29 years older than I was!

I took her to the airport, a 2 ½ hour drive to Nashville, a drive I never minded because it gave me an excuse to shop and eat. After I dropped her off, I had a mocha, a Starbucks treat, and stopped by Target to shop. While there, I ended up purchasing a giant Toblerone candy bar. On the way home I ate the entire Toblerone. I had already consumed other chocolates, fast food, and additional high caloric atrocities. I was shocked by my own behavior. How could I have eaten an entire Toblerone? The big Toblerone. By myself?

Why did this behavior distress me? It's not like I wasn't used to eating ridiculous amounts of food. Inordinate consumption was a way of life for me. I was disgusted with myself, as was often the case, with the amount and kinds of food I ate, usually in secret. The next morning, I determined to change.

I woke up. It was a new day, a day full of possibility. I decided to exercise. Being so out of shape, the logical course of action was to take a walk. I knew I wouldn't be able to go far. That was really frustrating because about two years before I was in (relatively) good shape, at least for 6 months. Oh well, I thought, this time is going to be different. Even though I had uttered those words countless times, I somehow, despite my past, believed it to be true.

I put my baby in the stroller, and off we went. I made it to the primary school in my town, not too far, but a start. When I came home, I got on the scale. 194.6 pounds. Ugh. This was not the first time I'd been in the mid 190s. The last time I lost weight I started around 185. So, not only did I regain all that I lost, but I also added about 10 pounds to the mix.

I decided to go on a diet, but only for the day. I became aware that all I had was today, June 5. That was the only day I had. My motto became "just today."

Just today. It didn't matter that every other diet I had tried I failed. It didn't matter that I was likely to fail at this diet. It didn't matter that I could maybe only eat better this one day. All I had was June 5. That was it, the only day I had to worry about. All the other days of my life, my triumphs and my failures were gone. I chose not to live in the shadow of what may happen tomorrow. I therefore chose to exercise and eat well for that day.

I would eat the Weight Watchers way, through the point system yet again. I didn't sign up this time because I already knew the system and had saved most of the literature.

With Weight Watchers you are allowed so many points in a day based on your current weight. On my self-modified Weight Watchers program, I decided 1 point was roughly 50 calories. The point system considers fat grams and dietary fiber too. In the past, while on Weight Watchers, I would usually stay within my given points for a day. The system recommends so many fruits, vegetables, and dairy products per day; recommendations I always ignored. I felt I was doing well to simply significantly reduce my caloric intake. I would eat sensibly most of the time, but always reserved points for treats. My husband likes to eat ice cream at night and so do I. I also love getting the other variety of "diet" desserts like fudgesicles, and low-fat Twinkie-like cakes.

I told myself it was simply ridiculous to think of living a life without sweets, so I needed to incorporate them into my new eating lifestyle. To eliminate sweets, even while on a diet, seemed impossible, unrealistic, immoderate, and even unhealthy (psychologically).

This time around I decided I would take the Weight Watchers recommendations for fruits and vegetables seriously. I needed to make a real difference in my lifestyle if there was going to be any possibility of losing and sustaining the weight loss. I knew I could lose weight but had *no* confidence in my abilities to maintain it.

I had heard of people being on diets and claiming to be *full*. I was only ever full when operating unleashed from reason's constraints and therefore "free" to eat as much of whatever I wanted. What if I ate lots of vegetables … what would that do to me? Would I be satisfied? Is that even possible? I would find out.

This time I would attempt to eat in a well-balanced way. I decided to not banish treats as a possibility, but plan on not having any today. I would tell myself every morning that today I would not eat wedding cake, just today. Tomorrow I might make a different decision. Tomorrow was tomorrow, who knows what the future may bring? Today, June 5; however, I planned to eat in a manner that was conducive to a healthy life, a peaceful less frenetic life.

June 5 passed. At the end of the day, I'd made it; I exercised and ate balanced meals.

June 6, I got up, got the baby ready and out the door we went. Again, I talked to myself about *this* day, the only day I had. Who cares what I did yesterday or what tomorrow holds? The food sins of my past were not going to determine my choices for this day. Tomorrow I might run to Wal-Mart in the morning, purchase five chocolate glazed donuts and devour them in the privacy of my car. Who knows? Today; however, I would not eat the donuts. Today I would eat in a moderate fashion. I was the one in control of the day. Not my past, not my future. June 6 was present to me.

What the post-enlightenment philosopher Blasé Pascal said about the importance of focusing on the present resonated with me:

> We do not rest satisfied with the present. We anticipate the future as too slow in coming, as if in order to hasten its course; or we recall the past, to stop its too rapid flight. So imprudent are we that we wander in the times which are not ours and do not think of the only one which belongs to us; and so idle are we that we dream of those times which are no more and thoughtlessly overlook that which alone exists. For the present is generally painful to us. We conceal it from our sight, because it troubles us; and, if it be delightful to us, we regret to see it pass away. We try to sustain it by the future and think of arranging matters which are not in our power, for a time which we have no certainty of reaching.
>
> Let each one examine his thoughts, and he will find them all occupied with the past and the future. We scarcely ever think of the present; and if we think of it, it is only to take light from it to arrange the future. The present is never our end. The past and the present are our means; the future alone is our end. So we never live, but we hope to live; and, as we are always preparing to be happy, it is inevitable we should never be so. (Pascal, *Pensees*, no. 172)

June 6 passed. All of June, July, August, and September too. Each and every day I chose to live in the present, to make healthy choices for the day. As each day came and went, I found it was not too difficult. I focused, especially in the beginning, on making certain I ate at least five times a day.

For breakfast I'd have a SlimFast. What I love about SlimFast is its tastiness and that it is contained and pre-measured. I have never once had a SlimFast and been tempted to have another. SlimFast, for me, is filling and does not leave me with the desire to gorge myself. Cereal, on the other hand, is one of my many food nemeses. Could I ever eat enough Honey Bunches of Oats? Enough Cheerios? I love to eat bowl after bowl of delicious fresh cereal with cold milk. You may be different. Chocolaty SlimFast may call your name.

I'd try to eat a snack around 10 a.m. before the effects of the SlimFast had completely worn off, usually a banana or apple. My favorite lunch was on Wednesdays. On Wednesdays I'd go to playgroup with my two youngest sons. After playgroup we'd go to McDonald's. Now, what is a girl on a diet who loves--and I mean *loves*--French fries doing at McDonald's? It just so happens they had a delicious Southwestern salad. I'd order it grilled without the sauce on the chicken and without the chips. It was fresh, yummy, good for me, and only 4 points!

The hardest food time of the day had always been in the afternoon, around 3 p.m. At this time I would either eat a piece of fruit, bread, a few hunks of cheese, or a scoop of peanut butter. For dinner I'd eat whatever my husband cooked. Christopher is an excellent cook. He is a very considerate cook, leaving out unnecessary butter, oil, cheese, and anything else that adds to girth. The year I began this change I started teaching full-time. Given our busy schedules, we ate out a lot.

After dinner I would be through with eating for the day. On the rare occasion I had not eaten enough points, I would have an apple, banana, or popcorn.

In addition to eating healthy foods and watching my portion sizes, I exercised regularly. Since I had three small children, worked full-time, and was involved in after work activities, I chose to exercise in the morning. I was a teacher and was therefore able to get up between 6 and 7 a.m. to exercise in the summer. When the school year started, I'd get up around 4:45 a.m. to go to the gym. I told myself at the time that I did not expect to be able (or even to desire) to get up this early in the long run. The long run did not matter. What mattered was today.

Every morning the alarm sounded, and I'd be up. Many times, I'd get up before the bell went off. I laid my workout clothes out the night before, so I wouldn't wake anyone else or give myself an excuse to skip the day. I tried to make myself take a day off occasionally, but, honestly, I didn't want to stay home in bed. I wanted to get up and go on a walk or to the gym.

From August, when I joined a local gym, to about November, I'd spend about 1 - 1 ½ hours in the morning exercising. I would walk to the gym down the street to do the elliptical or tread mill for about 35 to 40 minutes, work (lightly) on weights for another 10 to 15 minutes, do sit-ups and stretch for another 10 minutes, and then walk home. I loved my routine. I was starting to feel strong. I could see muscles in my legs! Exercising made me feel in control of myself.

It had been over three months. In the past, it was in the fourth month that my iron will began to shake, and my resolve began to slip. This time I began to fall off the healthy eating wagon in the fifth month.

October

We had lots of company that October. My husband's parents came to visit for a week and then my parents came for two weeks. My son had a mid-month birthday and Halloween candy was everywhere. I think it was the week before Halloween when I let candy become a part of my points system. It is insidious! You let a few bites through your teeth, and it all falls apart.

I started eating more.

Why do I overeat? Many reasons: stress, enjoyment, enjoyment, stress, because it's there, habit, for no discernible reason at all. It's hard to be in control of yourself when you feel fundamentally broken. The cracks are always there waiting to take over. It's hard to live for each day. It's hard, even when you're doing well.

That's a weird thing about losing weight. Despite the fact that I'd lost a bunch of weight, I was still essentially broken. I was trying to live and eat for each and every day. I was doing it, depriving myself just for that day. It is tiring to say no to yourself a million times a day, every day.

As it goes with an eating addiction, I found myself in a hole that was dug little by little. I did not take one bite of candy and throw all caution to the wind. Rather, I let it back in the door. Candy, treats, and sugar delights were now acceptable items to put in my daily food routine, as long as I stayed within (or close to) my points range.

As usual, the weight loss gave me a sense of over-confidence. I had controlled myself for this long, certainly a bit of candy couldn't hurt. This is what I told myself, and yet, at the same time, I knew I was lying. Socrates' motto was "know thyself." My entire diet past is littered with good attempts and achievements shattered by the very innocent-looking candy bar, the scoop of light ice cream, the piece of layered cake.

I was now eating sweets, but I tried my best to eat out in the open, to not hide. I was so used to eating damaging food by myself so no one would see what I was doing. Hiding. I didn't want to hide my aberrant behavior, but I was still embarrassed and ashamed.

By late October/early November, I had lost almost 40 pounds! I was in the 150s! I felt great in my clothes. I had not spent much on a new wardrobe so far, because I did not want to stay in the 150s. My goal was to have my BMI in the healthy range. I had already moved from *morbidly obese* to *obese* to *overweight*, but I wanted to be in the normal weight BMI category, which, given my height tops out at 131.9 pounds.

November and December, the party season

I continued to exercise rigorously. I continued to count points, but not as religiously. So many temptations, so much good food. It was the party season, you know. Why not feast?

By the end of December, I weighed 155 pounds. Even though I was not being as careful as I had been in the fall, I was still making progress. I was still exercising. I was still trying to shock myself back to reality by thinking of the calories in the Snickers bar I had last night vs. the energy I was exerting on the elliptical machine that morning. As much as I worked out in the morning, I was barely able to work off one of the treats I consumed the day before, and there were usually many treats for which I needed to atone. At least I was still trying.

In every other attempt I had made to lose weight, once I started down the slippery slope of eating sweets and larger portions, my exercising would decrease until I was back to my old patterns of overeating and inactivity. This time, for some unknown reason, I kept on exercising. My conscience kept talking to me, telling me to limit the sweets.

But I felt like a grave digger. I was digging my own grave and dragging myself back to the bleakness of my compulsions. I saw my trajectory and I wanted to change it. On numerous occasions I would say to myself, "Something is going to change. I won't be taken back to the size 18+, XL wardrobe. Something must change. What will it be? God, please send me help!"

As the winter progressed, I slipped back into my old eating patterns. In January, I started going to a lovely coffee shop and working on my classes there. I liked getting away from my home and office. The coffee shop was warm and inviting.

I'm not a big coffee drinker, but I'll drink just about anything you can add chocolate to. While there I would get a 12 oz non-fat, no-whip mocha. I figured this was about 4 points, and I was getting a milk product in. I then discovered the latté. This was even better. Only 2 points, no chocolate though. After a few weeks I decided I did in fact need a bit of chocolate to go with my yummy coffee, so I bought two small chocolate covered caramel truffles.

My rationale? I told myself I was spending the extra time and money to go to the coffee shop because I deserved a break, an environment that was peaceful and relaxing to work in. This is true. But I was lying; I was there for the sweets.

This combination of truffles and coffee continued for a few weeks. Then one day I added one chocolate chip cookie. The barista asked if I wanted it heated. Yes! There I sat, my 2-point latté and my mystery point cookie. Delicious.

Over the next few months, I visited the coffee shop as much as I could. I live in a small town; the coffee shop was in the next town over, about a 15-20 minute drive. I taught on Tuesdays and Thursdays, so I couldn't go then, but most Monday, Wednesday, and Friday mornings I was there. Sometimes I would justify the drive by noting it was good to get out of town, or by not drinking a SlimFast for breakfast I could have my latte and cookie (which by the way was now *two* cookies).

I had still not thrown *all* caution to the wind. I tried to find out how many calories were in these hideously delicious cookies. After a few emails to the cookie company and phone calls to the coffee shop, I found out: 360 calories per cookie! That's 7 points per cookie! That means my little breakfast of coffee and cookies added up to 16 points! I was only supposed to eat about 23 points a day.

I was glad, and not glad, to find out the truth about my indulgences. Every morning on the way to the gym I would tell myself that today I would not go to the coffee shop. Not today. All I had was today and today I could live without coffee and sweets. I tried (unsuccessfully) to re-convince myself of this every day, not just Monday, Wednesday, and Friday, because I finally visited the coffee shop on my campus.

The Skyhawk café was small but had what I wanted. A latté, but not with non-fat milk, and one of the best desserts of all – GIANT Rice Krispies Treats. For a couple of months, most Tuesdays and Thursdays I'd get a latte or mocha and a rice crispy treat. On Thursdays I'd have lunch with my husband at our favorite Mexican restaurant. All fall I was able to resist the chip bowl at La Canasta, but no longer.

I was in an oh-so-familiar spiral. Little by little my willpower faded. Eating a treat (or multiple treats) here or there, larger portions, ice cream at night with my husband. Easter rolled around and I found myself hoarding and hiding my two favorite Easter candies, Cadbury Eggs and Reese's Peanut Butter Eggs. I bought so many Cadbury eggs. I have no idea how many. I was up to eating about four a day. I was in an almost perpetual bad mood, was tired, and back to being hooked on sugar.

To illustrate how irrational I was becoming, it wasn't just myself I was taking to the coffee shop. It started on a Friday, a mommy/son day. I thought it would be a special treat to take my son to the coffee shop with me. My plan was to take him there, read books, play Uno and, of course, get my latté and cookies. I knew he would want a cookie, and that was fine with me because it meant I could indulge too.

This became a habit in which I would drive to the coffee shop whenever I could, usually going through the drive-thru with two kids in tow for "breakfast." Yes, I let my five-year-old son eat chocolate chip cookies and drink Sprite for breakfast just so I could indulge my selfish, immoderate food desires. That kind of behavior is seriously disordered and self-centered. Being run by my belly and passions at the expense of others – my own children!

This was not the first time these destructive food habits affected my children. Before I started this latest diet, I would regularly recommend going to Dairy Queen, Sonic, or McDonalds, not out of a concern for the kids, but so I could get my sugar/unhealthy food fix. It is a terrible thing to be controlled by your emotions and not your reason.

Though slipping back, I wasn't totally in the pit of gluttonous despair yet. Although the bonds of sugar addiction closed around me, I still had a glimmer of hope. I had not stopped exercising, though it was now only three to four times a week. This was something unusual. I had been exercising from June 2009 to April 2010. Eleven months!

Something had to change. I'd gained about five pounds and knew if I couldn't get control of the sugar situation I would go completely back to old habits.

People at church, at work, and friends were coming up to me, complementing me on how good I looked, what a great job I was doing. "Merry you look so good, so different." I had to constantly fight the urge to confess, "I don't deserve this body. I don't deserve to have lost these 40 pounds. Do you know what I'm eating right now? Do you know I'm not counting my points? Do you know, do you know I'm sneaking food? Don't praise me, don't praise me." Instead, I would just smile and say, "Thank you." I felt so inauthentic.

To be consumed by food. To be obsessed with food. To be twisted up in knots. To have a good day or bad day dependent on what you eat. This is no life. This is no way to live. Yet that was my life. This is my addiction. I have disordered desires when it comes to food. What could I do about this hopeless looking situation?

I had forgotten about living for the day. Or more, I felt powerless to say, "NO," to my own inordinate passions. I was embarrassed, moody, and erratic. I wanted to be freed. *Tomorrow* no mochas, no lattés, no marshmallow treats. It's horrid, fighting against your nature, endlessly. It's a miserable way to exist, and I was indeed miserable.

How did I get back in the pit? Sugar. Sugar calls my name. The sirens call. Once I let sugar in, I caved to all my food wishes.

I read books and books on dieting. How to do it? How to overcome? I had to find something that would work for me.

What was going to happen now? This was the same pattern I'd been through my entire life, loss and gain, loss and gain. I did not want to go back. I was embarrassed to go back, admit defeat. What could possibly change? Could I really change?

Chapter 3: My Last Diet Ever, Really

I have put off writing this book because I'm a private person. I don't like being vulnerable. What I have to tell you about my last diet is embarrassing to me, but the truth, nonetheless.

My diet was in rapid failure. I was falling apart and looking for a lifeline. My eating habits were shot, and I was gaining weight. I was praying and looking for a lifeline to save me from sinking into the pit of despair. Help came in the strangest way.

I was aware of the *Twilight* books, but not interested in them. I didn't read young adult fiction. The first movie was out, and I decided to see it. I was hooked and immediately read the books.

You know, life is mysterious. That something speaks to one person and means nothing to another is the way of the universe. I was open, searching for help. While reading Meyer's books I had an epiphany. I was a sugar addict and the only way to be truly free was to cut out sugar, completely, forever. That was the solution to my eating problems. I was a sugar addict. Therefore, no more sugar for me. Ever.

It's not an exaggeration to admit I truly thought my life had changed forever. I was free … or so I thought.

I gave up sugar forever and was back in the game! I was eating right again, ramped up my exercise to everyday, created a diet club for my friends and wrote a diet book about how to permanently lose weight through a virtue ethical[6] approach to eating.

---

[6] Virtue ethics is a philosophical way to think about how people should behave. The focus is on becoming a virtue person through continually practicing and acting excellent in every situation. More on this in Section III.

And guess what happened? The same as always. Through the summer and into early winter I was high on my new dieting epiphany! But then it all unraveled.

The difference this time was that I genuinely thought I was cured of my food addiction. I sincerely thought I had beaten my food demon. When I fell off the wagon again, I was utterly shattered.

To understand how bad I fell, here is an excerpt from the diet book I wrote that, thankfully, was never published. The following passage illustrates how convinced I was that I was cured:

Finding Virtue

My philosophy courses introduce undergraduates to philosophy and ethics. I'm a virtue ethicist of sorts and am convinced the only way to have a good life is to live in a virtuous way. I don't always measure up, but I am certain the only way to live a truly human life is to live a virtuous life.

Think about it. What is the alternative to seeking after virtue? Vice, viciousness. What is the alternative to seeking after the cardinal virtues of wisdom, courage, moderation, and justice? Only through pursuing virtue do any of us stand a chance of living a flourishing life.

An excellent way to understand the virtuous life is through finding role models. When we see someone acting in a virtuous way, it shows us possible paths. It shows us what we could do too. Role models can be found in many places from literature to movies to historical figures to parents, friends, and others we know.

The idea behind having role models is not that we do exactly what they do, but rather it helps us to navigate life's circumstances as we build our own moral reserves. When we see what others have done, what they have accomplished, it can inspire us to push beyond our preconceived boundaries to do what we thought was impossible, or unlikely.

When I read the *Twilight* series, I was struck by the commitment Carlisle and his family had to the virtuous life. Carlisle was given a nature that was an abomination, and yet, in the face of despair, he found a way out.

Carlisle was fundamentally changed, against his will, so that his natural inclinations became vicious. Despite his intense drive for human blood, he fought against who he had become. He fought to find a different way and he succeeded. Carlisle is the picture of a virtuous man. He is wise, moderate, courageous, just, compassionate, forgiving, accepting of others, and full of hope and love.

Does it sound strange to praise Carlisle as a role model for human behavior when he is first of all fictitious and secondly, not even a human but a vampire? Literature is full of wonderful characters to admire and learn from. I felt this way when I read *Jane Eyre*. What a woman of uncompromising virtue! And what of Sam and Frodo from *The Lord of the Rings*? They are hobbits who have so much to teach us about friendship, courage, and what is worth fighting for.

I was struggling with my weight issues, falling back into desolation. It was at this time I read the *Twilight* books and was shown another way. The vampires in the Cullen family had dietary issues and so do I. They had to fight against their nature to be better than they were. I had to fight against my nature if I was going to get out from this crushing despair of the unending diet cycle.

The difference between the Cullens and me was that they were winning their fight and I was losing. I wanted to be like the Cullens. I wanted to stand up to my lustful ways and say, "ENOUGH! NO MORE! I will not be controlled by my passions any longer."

Was this going to be hard? Yes. Was it going to cost me? Dearly, but it was hard for the Cullens too, in many ways, and look at the rewards their lifestyle brought them: peace, love, and family.

What was it going to cost me? Well, a large part of my life was centered around food. I was, in some ways, living to eat - not eating to live. I was obsessed with food – making sure I could get my fix. What would my life be like if I just ate "tofu"? If I gave up on food as a source of pleasure and recreation, what would I do? If I were serious about changing, the price was going to be **high.** I always imagined the real price for this kind of change was too high, not within my psychological reserves to pay.

Of all the diets I had been on, I had never given up desserts or diet soda. How could I? Having daily sweets was akin to breathing air. The very thought of giving up desserts was an anathema to me, for I didn't want to live without them, indeed, I didn't think it was even *possible*.

The third day into reading about the Cullens I decided to change, to eat "tofu," to eat to live. I was no longer going to be concerned with the tastiness of my meals, but rather that my meals sustained my bodily existence. I decided no snacking, no treats at all ... ever.

The first three weeks of my sustainability project went rather smoothly. At times I was irritated because I was hungry, but I pushed through. I enjoyed this new sensation called hunger. I had rarely allowed myself to be hungry. I told myself it was okay to be hungry. Get used to it.

As the weeks progressed, I began having a harder time with meal choices. I was eating a bit too much at mealtime and was upset by my lack of self-control. As it goes with new ventures, eventually it's not new anymore and you are stuck with living the plan in all its hideous monotony.

In the beginning I remembered the desire to be challenged! I wanted to be tempted by food and say no. I felt so sure of myself. I had changed and I knew it. I was so confident and desired to be tempted, even though I knew the time was coming when real temptation would be waiting for me.

About three weeks into my no snacking, no treats plan, I got hungry. I was tempted. Instead of meeting my temptation head on and with glee as I anticipated, I was lambasted with the force and relentless character of my tempter. Food temptation is my constant companion. A real thorn in my flesh that won't go away. I'm usually fine in the morning. Okay before lunch and bullied from mid-day until I decide to go to bed.

Last night it was just one more tablespoon of peanut butter. Just one more piece of low-calorie bread. I'd eaten dinner. I had a bit after dinner because I needed to eat a little more to reach my calorie intake goal for the day. This little bit afterward became a full-blown battle. My tempter told me over and over of the pleasure of peanut butter and the softness and comfort the bread had to offer. This put me in a sour mood. My husband thought I was mad at him. I wasn't mad at him; I was preoccupied with the internal struggle in my head:

Tempter: But it tastes so good!

Reason: It does taste good, but one more won't leave me satisfied.

Tempter: You won't know unless you try.

Reason: I've tried my whole life to be satisfied by food, and I always want more.

Tempter: (new tactic) Well, one more won't hurt anything, don't be such a control freak!

Reason: If I'm a control freak it's your fault! You have no control, no ability to be satiated. One more will lead to another, and another and I am not willing to spend 500 extra calories on peanut butter and bread tonight!

Repeat this conversation over and over for a few hours and you'll get the picture.

Temptation lurks around us all, waiting for us, regardless of our personal issues. The Cullens fight hard to be freed from their blood lust. They were winning their battle and I was enslaved. What did the Cullens have that I lacked? How could they deny themselves pleasure and I always gave in?

And so, I gave up sugar. I talked to it like it was a real enemy. Anyone around me at that time would get an earful of my new way of life. No sugar. One of my favorite lines was, "There's no good that can come from that." I remember thinking I was in an actual, literal war. Me against sugar. And I knew I'd win.

I therefore cannot just listen to my body for the cues I need to stop eating. I must instead go against 25 years of physical and mental conditioning and listen to what my reason tells me. This is a fight. A fight I am determined to win – with God's help.

Fight the fight. Who wants to be at war? No one. If you have food issues and you don't fight, you are living under an unjust dictator. You are allowing yourself to be held hostage to the irrational demands of your body. Take up arms and fight. Remember, "no justice, no peace." The weapons in this war are the virtues. You are worth the fight. Your life, the way in which you want to live – YOUR FREEDOM – is worth it. Arm yourself and diligently fight your passions. In the end, if you stand firm, you will win.

I now fight each day. I wish I could tell you once you get into a rhythm it's not so bad. That is a lie. You know how you can tell it is a lie? Yo-yo dieting. No one who loses 30, 50, 100 pounds plus thinks they will cave and gain it back. The truth about weight loss is that most of it is temporary.

If you are intent on losing weight and keeping it off, you must wake every morning ready to fight. Some days are harder than others. Expect to be continually assaulted with temptations for their tentacles are rooted deep within. Regardless of what comes your way choose this day to not give up or give in. Choose to fight!

You're in the fray. Bombs are coming at you (you pass by a bakery), machine guns are firing (you go out to lunch with co-workers), tear gas is thrown in your bunker (it's Halloween!); how do you survive?

***

As you can see from this excerpt, I was under the false assumption that my weight issues and battle were between an outside temptation and my strength of resolve. The issue was that of willpower. That was the only way to win.

I wrote a 300-page diet book on how thinking and practicing the virtues could free you from yo-yo dieting and help you make peace with food. I felt so insanely free. This demon of food addiction I'd carried for decades was gone forever! I wanted to share what I'd found, how I'd broken free, with the world. I couldn't wait to go on *Oprah* with my newly published book to help all those who had suffered like me.

Unfortunately, I was in denial. I was wound so tight; it seems the snap that came was inevitable. But I couldn't see it. I couldn't see the extreme control I had over my food wasn't sustainable or even real.[7]

Months before I completely fell apart and went headlong into BED, I binged and purged for a few weeks[8], but I couldn't see I was tumbling out of control. I wouldn't allow myself to see what was right before my eyes, and I suffered for my blindness.

---

[7] Take a look at Appendix C, which is 30 days of my food diet journal from the summer of 2009. That is not the picture of someone who had really won anything. I've included this specifically for those of you who have not had an eating disorder. We all desire to be understood. I hope to show the mental anxiety and energy an eating disorder drains out of a person.

[8] See Appendix D

Chapter 4: The Great Falling Apart that Led to the Dawn

I sent my Virtue Diet manuscript to a few literary agents and had a promising interaction with one. She liked my book but said it's typical to have a two-year weight-loss success track record before publishing a book like this. She said I should contact her in six months. Six months, I could wait.

As I was waiting for the months to pass, I thought all was going fine with me, mentally. I was free, never to return to the old me.

Instead, I crashed and burned.

I still don't really understand what happened the day my no-dessert resolve ended. Nothing out of the ordinary had happened. It was around Christmas, and I had ordered See's Candy (the best in the world) for presents and had a box or two in my closet.

For some reason I decided to open a box and have some. Why? Why would I do this? I hadn't eaten a dessert in nine months, and I was cured. Wasn't I?

Well, I ate.

Was devastated!

And just like that, sugar was back in my life.

I started eating too much, behind closed doors, ashamed. I worked on editing my virtue dieting book in-between eating and purging. Yeah, that was back too.

I remember taking a weekend trip to get away and edit the book, while eating copious amounts of fast food and laughing/crying at the irony.

When the literary agent ended up passing on my book, I was relieved. I could just give up.

And so I ate. I ate so much and couldn't stop.

I went through drive-thrus and stuffed the fries in my face while sitting in my car, crying. Have you ever eaten while you're crying? It's not pleasant.

The following year and a half were a blur.

I ended up in therapy, on anti-depressants, and was diagnosed with binge eating disorder.

The weight slowly, but steadily, returned. I had a hard time getting out of bed. Since I'm a hider, I was able to plaster on a smile and teach my classes. But on the days I wasn't teaching and home alone with my toddler, I'd put on another video for him to watch as I pulled the covers over my head while crying, because I felt I was messing him up. What he'd remember from his early formative years was a mother who did nothing with him.

I barely functioned, but I did. I met my obligations, and a little more. I started writing a young adult fiction novel because I thought if I were writing I couldn't eat. Ha! Turns out you can eat and type at the same time.

The hardest part, by far, of this awful experience was the deep and abiding sense of disappointment. I had never been so disappointed in my life. I had utterly convinced myself I was free from the addiction of sugar, from the tyranny of food. I was free. I'd not felt that freedom before. I was completely certain I'd beaten my addiction.

The disappointment was breathtaking and vast. It filled every part of me. I walked around, feeling like the wind had been knocked out of my lungs. I've never experienced anything so all-encompassing before or since. My disappointment was a constant haunting. More than the throb of a headache that won't let you forget its presence. I felt swallowed whole. While it was my constant, unrelenting companion for well over a year, some moments were unbearable. I was a woman caught in the grips of despair and denial. This couldn't be happening to me.

As I sit here now, almost a decade away from the crushing despair, it's hard even for me to understand it. I mean, come on, a failed diet. Boo-hoo. It's not like someone died. Or even had a severe illness. What was the big deal?

I think I was done with myself. I could no longer count on myself. It was self-betrayal. I was unmoored and couldn't right myself. I'd put all my eggs in this basket; the basket of fighting my Sugar Demon and winning! I thought I had won the hardest fight of my life. And I fought. I planned and plotted.

I remember being in the social hall of my church and having a conversation with a very nice woman. She complemented me on my weight loss. She went on to tell me she didn't understand why people were overweight. What she did was watched what she ate. For instance, she brings yogurt to work for lunch and eats a sensible diet.

She was trying to connect with me, which I appreciated. How could she know that I was on the downward spiral? How could she know I'd binged earlier that day? All she could see was my outsides, I'd lost weight. Good job, Merry!

All I felt was the fraud I was. I wanted to set her straight, tell her she was so wrong about me and many others who are overweight. But how could I? I assessed she had not the time nor interest to know the truth. And I certainly wasn't able to tell the truth. I was dumbfounded by my actions. Too ashamed. In retrospect, I hope I sold the good intentioned woman short. I hope if I had told her why she was wrong to say all overweight people had a simple problem of eating too much, she would see her error.

But the haze of despair and disappointment had already taken me. I couldn't accept what was happening to me. It felt like it was being done to me, instead of me being the perpetrator. I see why the old religion of Manichaeism was popular. Manichaeism taught there were two powerful gods – the god of darkness and the god of light – who are locked in an eternal battle. People are made of both gods. When I do something bad, it's not really "me," but the god of darkness. The classic cry of, "the devil made me do it."

It felt like it wasn't me, but it was, which made it worse. I was the one who stuck a knife in my chest. I was the robber. Why would I abandon myself? How could I do that to myself? I still don't understand. How could this have happened? I did everything right:

I talked to my food. I told it why it was bad and could no longer have me. I was free!

I blogged.

I played mind games.

I formed a weight-loss group, comprised of friends, the Existential Eaters Society.

I wrote a weight-loss book to share the good news. *I am free and you can be too.*

But it was all empty lies. I was not free. I was self-deceived. *But I was positive I was free.*

The disappointment enveloped me, accusing me on endless loop. How could I have allowed this to happen? Why did I give in? How could I have ultimately lost? I went in and out of denial as I binged. I didn't really look in a mirror for the rest of that year.

Binge eating disorder isn't rational. It isn't overeating. When well-meaning people treat it as such, it stings. It's arresting when people think BED is just eating too much at dinner, or the occasional entire pizza. We all know how it feels to be misunderstood. I am certainly guilty of looking at others and funneling their behavior through my lens of experience and knowledge.

It wasn't until I came to terms with my deep disappointment with myself that I began to heal.

I fantasized about checking myself into an eating disorder facility. I searched the internet for the ones closest to me, seriously considered the financial cost, but the family cost was always too high for me. I was unwilling to get the help I needed because, when did I have the time? I worked. My husband worked. We had three kids. How could I get away for a month or two? No, not feasible. But that didn't keep me from daydreaming of being in a hospital room where people brought me food. The right amount of food. Where I didn't have to make any food decisions. Where I didn't have to shop for it, feed it to others, gather around it, make decisions about it. In my mind, I built checking myself in for care into a great big fantasy, where I could finally pull the covers over my head for a long time without disappointing anyone.

A year and a half passed in a blur. I half functioned, gutted. I still worked, wrote, went to church, tried to love my family.

I had been on anti-depressants for about a year when I decided I didn't need them anymore. I was wrong, and went right back on. Six months after that, in the summer of 2011, the sun came out.

Christopher and I decided to take the kids on a massive three-week camping trip from our home in Tennessee to visit my sister and her then boyfriend (now husband) in Seattle. Tent camping the entire way.

I'd call this camping trip a bit ambitious since our family had not been camping together before.

Our first night out it rained and soaked the tent. We were up at 2 a.m. at the camp site laundry mat, running through our supply of quarters.

We continued to be plagued by rain, and had the time of our lives. We camped a week out there, staying at cute little KOAs and the like. We rented a house for a week in Seattle, and camped our way back, spending a few days in Yellowstone.

We played loads of mini golf, slept in tents on the ground, our youngest learned to swim, and saw much of this great nation.

Somewhere along this trip, and I honestly can't recall when, I decided I didn't need the anti-depressants.

I was a bit leery of stopping them since I certainly wasn't ready six months prior. But something about the trip helped me begin to let go.

I have loads of flaws and regrets, but one of the hardest things I've ever had to do was letting myself off the hook. I had deeply betrayed myself. I was so disappointed in my own behavior. The disappointment hung about my head and rang in my ears on a loop.

But it was over. I'd lost. I had to accept it.

I had told myself I was in a war with food, with sugar specifically. I had to fight, constantly. But that wasn't what I really thought. I thought the war was over and I had won.

Hubris.

I had lost, and I had to accept it. The fact that I gained weight back was not the issue. I'd been a yo-yo dieter for twenty-five years. But I really, genuinely, thought I conquered my eating addiction.

The key, for me, to recovering from BED was accepting defeat, forgiving myself, recognizing I was (and will always be) a food addict, and allowing myself to eat whatever I wanted.

SECTION II: OVERCOMING BINGE EATING DISORDER

Chapter 5: How I Overcame Binge Eating Disorder

To be crystal clear, this is my story of recovery. This is what worked for me. I am not a doctor, and I am not a nutritionist. I am a woman who has been on this journey for over thirty years. And what I have to say is not easy to hear because it is not a quick-fix program and it's not a story of how a person conquers all her demons, and in the process loses unwanted weight forever!

No, that is not my story. I am still a food addict and overweight. But what I did lose is the control food had over me and I gained something priceless, peace with food.

In my quest to deal with BED, I read. I read and read all the books on weight-loss and eating disorders that looked interesting to me. So many good ideas. So many ideas I tried and failed at:

- Hey, girl, have you tried writing down everything you eat?[9]
- Hey, girl, have you tried writing down how you feel about everything you eat?
- Hey, girl, have you tried only eating when you sit at a table, alone, with only your food and no distractions?

What I realized is all this great food advice doesn't work for me because I'm obsessed with food. Thinking about food, to this day, makes me anxious. Thinking about it, planning it, taking stock of it, this is not for me.

---

[9] In this book I use feminine pronouns when referring to people in general. I by no means am trying to exclude men who find themselves with BED or an eating addiction.

When I was finally able to forgive myself for the massive disappointment of self-betrayal, I saw the only path that would never lead into the pit of eating despair was to head in the opposite direction, away from all diets and dieting mentality. To this end I came up with two personal rules:

#1 **No diets ever again**

#2 **No weighing ever again**

Something interesting happened. When I gave myself permission to eat what I wanted, I didn't want it so much. I think this only worked because I meant it. Truly meant it.

Have you ever met someone who wants to be in a romantic relationship, but hasn't found someone, so she or he is "taking a break" to work on herself instead? But you know it's just a game, and if the right person came around the corner, the "break" would be over.

No, this was not a psychological game I was playing with myself, and I knew it. Food has always played messed-up mind games with me, and I was done with it. Or trying to control it.

If you're an alcoholic, you give it up. Same with drugs.

But if you're a food addict, you don't get to do that. You must make peace with food. There is no other way.

My peace came in a white flag of surrender.

I overcame my binge eating disorder by giving up my desire for control. I stopped squeezing myself to death. I could never control the speed of the merry-go-round of my food-mind, so I just jumped off. Once I genuinely gave up on dieting and controlling the food I ate, I finally won.

The difference in winning this time was that the prize changed. I used to think "winning" was hitting my ideal weight and maintaining it.

I dumped that idea of winning for peace. When I sincerely gave up controlling my food intake, I won peace. I won freedom. I won a new outlook on what was important.

Chapter 6: The Trick

As I recovered from binge eating disorder, I discovered there was no trick to escape food addiction.

Shoot.

No magic pill or bargain to be made.

No psychological games.

The trick is there is no trick. There is no finagling out of food addiction. The only way out, I found, was to face myself and let go. Really, truly, completely let go of thinking my problems were:

1. I lacked self-control

2. The weight

These were not my problems. Not really. The problem is in my mind and brain.

Since I incorrectly diagnosed my problem for decades, my so-called solutions had me running in circles. I just had to find the right trick; the right wish, prayer, or diet and I could get control of myself and thereby be rid of the fat.

Finding the right trick to beat the fat brought about loads of daydreaming and magical thinking. For example, countless times, from the time I was a teenager to all too recently, I daydreamed of waking up thin. In the night, the weight fell off. It was a miracle! I tried to make it realistic by imagining waking in a bed oozing with my own fat – the fat that melted off. What a minuscule price to pay, waking up in the disgusting goo, to be free from the prison of fat.

I believe in miracles. I believed it was not outside the realm of possible events that this could happen for me.

I distinctly remember being at a philosophy conference and seeing a person suffering from morbid obesity, no longer able to walk from the crippling weight. I drifted from listening to the paper and being engaged in a sustained internal dialogue where I gifted this person my miracle. I wanted my fat gone, but this person needed the miracle more than I did.

I was years into my recovery when I had this hour-long conversation with myself and the gifting of my wish to him. Philosophy Conference Stranger, I wish you well.

What I came to realize, which set me on the journey of freedom from BED, is there is no trick. I knew there was no physical trick – weight loss surgery or pill – that would free me. I've always known it, kind of.

The trick I played was psychological. Psychological torment and denial.

With so many mind games I'd habituated myself to play, where to begin?

There's the, "I've eaten well today, I'm changed forever!"[10]

There's the classic, "Diet starts tomorrow, let's eat, drink, and be merry for tomorrow we **die**t."

As I search to explain the other constant games and destructive nihilistic self-talk, I find the sickness of my food addiction is like an ordering principle in my mind, in which my experience is (or was) constantly clouded. It was a way of everyday life, coloring all my experiences and encounters, whether food was present.

My food life was broken straight down the middle where food fell into one of two categories: good and bad. There were no neutral meals and snacks. I was always being good or bad, dependent on what and how much I ate. Every single day. A food was never a food. A salad was never a salad. A salad said

---

[10] This is a link to a video from College Humor that encapsulates how I felt many, many times when I said "no" to seconds or dessert https://www.youtube.com/watch?v=2pA78TnFvWI. Particularly in my youth, when I started a diet (day one or two), I was mad that I was still fat because I'd turned over a new eating-leaf! I shouldn't have to deal with my hugeness because that wasn't me anymore.

I was good. A salad for a meal? My mind would rejoice in my virtue, "You ate a salad – you're on a diet! Good work! It's about time. This time it's going to be different! Hip-hip hooray!!!"

When dieting, my mind never stopped. I thought if I could stay vigilant that would be the trick that would make this diet a success. When I was on a diet, I would constantly count calories (or points) – and I mean constantly. I'd add the calories for the day or meal, get lost in my brain, start again. I had the side constant banter of wondering if I was over or understating the truth of my consumption and start again. On a loop.[11]

Those of you with eating disorders know what I'm talking about. If you are not imagining a constant torrent of adding calories and picking through every eating choice, I'm happy for you.

When I was dieting, there was the eating and waiting to eat again. I mean, sitting and thinking incessantly about the next thing I could eat – all the while "knowing" I don't deserve to eat anything. *Eating makes you fat. Fat is the worst thing ever. Don't eat as long as you can take it.* This disordered self-talk fed into overeating because I was starving physically and mentally.

My recovery from binge eating disorder began when I let go. I used to try to hide my sick thoughts from myself because I knew they were false and seriously disturbed. I'd push them to the back of my mind, where they played on a loop.

---

[11] For a very long time I wrote down everything I ate. I turned everything I ate into a Weight Watcher's point or calorie/fat/fiber running total. For years, I dutifully carried the WW's little book with me where I recorded all my food and dieting behavior. I haven't used food consumption tracking apps much, which I'm sure many of you have. Food apps are blessings to some and curses for others. For me, they were a curse that fed my addiction. They were growing in popularity as I entered my food addiction recovery. Thankfully, I didn't use them much.

The trick, I finally found, was there really was no trick. There was no way to find the "right" way to win against the food addiction.

I had to let go of the idea of finding the right trick and accept the facts:

- I am, and will always be, a food addict.
- I will not be the 'thin' me I longed for.

About a year and a half after my Last Diet Ever, I found life went on. The kids were still being parented. My husband was still there loving me. My friends hadn't changed. My job was still my job.

The crushing disappointment from my diet failure lessened. I had to accept it. This began my reconciliation process to myself.

In the midst of depression and BED, I explored recovery options. I went to a counselor regularly. I was on antidepressants. I read about BED. I went on a spiritual retreat.

Eventually, I let go. Gradually. It didn't happen overnight.

But, looking back, apart from managing the depression, the most significant part of my recovery was letting go.

Letting go of the crushing self-disappointment for not being 'strong enough' to set myself free from my food addiction.

When I let go of the demoralizing disappointment, I also gave up the dream of being normal weight. Really let it go.

Letting go meant no more psychological tricks. I realized this meant I could no longer restrict or monitor my food intake. At all. This idea came about organically and seemed quite reasonable. It wasn't scary, it wasn't freeing at first either, but it seemed the only thing left to do. Accept, give up, and move forward.

From the outside, it was an extreme reaction to a "failed diet." Yet another misunderstanding of my mental illness.

Letting go set me on the path to freedom. I'd been bound for decades, ruled by the incessant banter and control of my internal food chatter.

Amazingly, since it was really, truly, not my goal anymore to lose weight, the noise in my head dropped off.

How? How could achieving a normal weight not be my goal anymore? Did I not know about the physical, social, and financial costs associated with obesity?

I know.

Then what?

Quality of life. My falling apart was a 'boundary situation' for me. A boundary situation is when we go through an event (it doesn't have to be traumatic), that shakes us so that we face the fact that we – no one else- decides what kind of life we live. We are the sum total of our choices.

I decided I'd rather be fat and sane than normal weight and insane.

Are those really the only two options, Merry? I mean, come on!

For me? Yes. And I have 30 years of evidence galore to back up my claim.

Why was I torturing myself? What was I really going to get from being normal weight? Would all of my problems magically disappear?

I finally believed being a smaller size was not the panacea I'd built it up to be. You know who didn't care what my weight was? My husband, my boys, my family, my friends. So why was I killing myself?

I did a cost/benefit analysis and decided I was better off not caring about food and weight. I found a new dream – a healthy mind.

I didn't want to waste any more of my life thinking about food.

So, I didn't.

While I gave up on dieting, the scars were deeply etched in my psyche.[12] I developed PTSD about dieting. The thought of watching my food intake was painful. Not only would the memory of my Last Diet Ever send me into a panic, but hearing someone go on a diet made me flinch, internally feeling, *Why would you do that to yourself? Don't you know you're going to fail? I'm so sorry for you! I'm so sorry you are going through the cycle. I hope it doesn't last long. Peace to you.*

This is not me being cynical. This is not me saying, "I couldn't do it so neither can you." This is a recognition of food disorders being just that – disorders. Do you know people have the same small chance (5% to 20%, depending on the study) of sustaining long-term weight loss as someone does beating a heroin addiction? DO YOU HEAR ME?

> THEN WHY ARE WE TELLING PEOPLE TO LOSE WEIGHT ON THEIR OWN? AND WHEN THEY DON'T LOSE WEIGHT, WE TELL THEM THEY ARE WEAK AND THERE IS SOMETHING MORALLY WRONG WITH THEM? THIS MUST CHANGE.

I overcame BED by giving up on mind tricks and replacing the sick thinking with not thinking about food. Instead, I ate what I wanted when I wanted.

When I did this, when I gave myself permission – true permission – free of mind games and judgement – or even

---

[12] I don't want to paint a false picture of being free from dieting and binge eating disorder. Some days with food are still difficult. Sometimes I berate my body for its heft. Sometimes my mind does mental gymnastics about what and when to eat. But the noise seems to recede more and more. The disordered food talk is drying up, but it's not entirely gone. I don't expect it to be.

counting and noticing – to eat what I wanted, I stopped binging.

I haven't binged in nearly ten years.

Chapter 7: The Paradox

Hold up. How can I say that to overcome BED, eat what you want? Isn't that the problem, too much eating?

Eating too much is not the problem. The over consumption of food is the outward manifestation of an inward malady. (Again, let me be clear, I am not a doctor or psychologist. This is my story and what has worked for me. You – or the person you love who is suffering from BED – has an experience that is unique.)[13]

Once I decided to get off the cycle of dieting and join the team No Diet Ever, I meant it.

Contrary to dieting advice that tells you to empty your house of so-called "bad foods," I make certain these foods are readily available.

- M&M's in my underwear drawer? Check
- Ice cream in the freezer? Check
- Chips and other assortment of salty treats in the pantry? Check
- Full calorie soda in the refrigerator? Check.

For almost a decade now my house has had plenty of "no-no" foods. I have a rule about eating them. *Eat them.*

Eat them all! Buy whatever you want at the store! Go to the store or drive-thru when I have a craving.

In other words, scratch that itch!

---

[13] This is an important point. I am not an expert on BED or food addiction. I am, however, an expert on me. I am telling you what works for me. There are some people and some conditions in which it would be unwise to try what I've done. My best advice is to find a doctor/therapist/nutritionist who resonates with you. You have your own story and past. My overarching message is there is hope for you. Maybe my path will shed light on what *may* work for you. I encourage you to be active and creative as you recover from your eating disorder.

I know this sounds crazy. But mind games are all about restricting. The only way I found to stop the cycle of restriction was to not restrict. There are no foods or portions or locations off-limits.

I can eat whatever I want. And I genuinely mean it.

So, how much do I weigh?

I gained all the weight I lost in my Last Diet Ever.[14]

I believe this. I will never diet again. I will never restrict again.

How can this be? How could I really, straight faced, claim I will never diet again?[15] I'll tell you how. My real options are diet (restrict) and be mentally sick/incapacitated or not diet. There is no middle ground. If, at this point in this book, you don't believe me, I've done a poor job explaining what it's like for me and some others to live on a diet (restrictive mind set). If you need more evidence, see Appendix C for a look at what goes on in my mind when I restrict.

So, do I pig out regularly? No, not really. I could if I wanted to. I just find I don't want to or need to. Sure, I obviously eat more than I need to reach and maintain a healthy physical weight, but that is neither here nor there. I wanted out of my mental jail. That has become my priority.

---

[14] I was a stable weight for about seven years. About two years ago I began to gain weight, which I'll get to and has nothing to do with eating what I want.

[15] I want you to stop for just a moment. Stop what you are doing and imagine your life and what it would be like to never go on a diet again. Never. Ever. Never planning to go on one or feeling bad because you put it off again or just failed. Never restricting. Never going through your day or year thinking about good and bad foods. Can you imagine living this way? What would your life be like? Can you get your head around that kind of freedom?

If I am really free to eat whatever I want, someone like me who is a food addict, with sugar being my drug of choice … how does that really work?

You may be interested to know the Halloween candy in my house typically makes it well into the next holiday, usually bound for the trashcan sometime in the New Year.

When I let go of finding 'the trick' and truly gave myself the ability to eat whatever my heart desired, turns out my heart just didn't care as much.

A few days after Easter 2021, I was sitting by one of my kid's Easter baskets – most of the candy still in there. He'd gone back to college, leaving it. He didn't care about the candy. I looked through it and pulled out the chocolate bunny. My husband ate an ear. The next day I ate part of the body. The remnants of the half-eaten bunny remained on the coffee table by the rocking chair until I finally threw it out a week later.

A few days after the bunny made it to the trash, I tossed out the rest of my youngest son's basket. He'd picked out what he wanted.

Do my kids eat too much candy? Some of them do. Do I want that for them? No. What I don't want for them more is my eating disordered, diseased mindset. I am not their food police. I wish I were, but I think I would do more harm than good given my thirty years of food issues.

I realize this is less than ideal. But it is called facing facts. I am a food addict. I am a good mom in many ways, but I am not stellar when it comes to modeling a healthy relationship with food. Since I don't have a non-diseased way to deal with food, I decided long ago to let my kids be. I'm not saying my kids were raised on cotton candy, but my house has (obviously) not been the paragon of healthy eating 101.[16]

---

[16] I am not making light of the situation. I KNOW obesity is a serious issue. But I also know MENTAL ILLNESS sucks too. I picked my poison

So, we have crap snack food in the house. It hardly ever gets all the way eaten.

The only time I feel nervous is when I don't have the option of chocolate available to me. Looking back, and knowing it at the time too, when I am not in control of the food situation or feel that someone is watching me – I will overeat. I feel compelled to. Like a nervous tick.

The paradox is not binging by allowing myself to binge. Since I really, truly, psychologically unreservedly allow myself to binge, I have no need for it. It no longer serves its purpose.

This is how I made peace with food. This is how food became just food. There are no special, good, or bad foods. There is food. I can eat what I want. This is peace for me.

Questions to consider:
- What do you think would happen if you allowed yourself to eat what you wanted?
- What would it be like to never diet again?
- Would your quality of life increase or decrease if you decided to give up on dieting for the rest of your life?
- Imagine you have an infinite supply of the foods you binge on. Imagine as you ate, the foods just keep reappearing. Forever. With no end. Now imagine you gave yourself complete and utter permission to eat whatever you wanted whenever you wanted. What do you think would happen?

---

and try the best I can to encourage healthy eating for my kids, trying my best to not talk about food around them.

Chapter 8: Exercise

I 100% should exercise. All people should exercise regularly, as they are able. We should exercise because we have physical bodies. It turns out our bodies work better, feel better, and last longer when we have a habit of exercising.

This is not news. It is certainly not news to those who have lived their life on a diet.

For me as for many with food addictions, exercise and dieting go hand-in-hand. If I was dieting, I was exercising. Without exception.

I always saw exercise as a necessary part of losing weight. Why in the world would I torment myself on a diet and make it take longer than necessary? That doesn't make any sense. If you exercise, you get rid of the weight faster.

Some people exercise and feel better afterwards. This rarely was the case for me, even after exercising continuously over a long period of time. However, on my Last Diet Ever, I did enjoy walking in nature and aerobics. Exercise is not all drudgery, but I've never experienced the runner's high. The only high I found was when the scale showed I lost weight.

Exercising to lose weight colors the experience. The goal is not health, but a certain body type. It was demoralizing to be often reminded an hour on the treadmill wasn't enough to counter-act the treat I already ate.

For this reason, I have a mixed relationship with exercising. It's hard for me, now, to exercise without bringing food into the mental equation.

For years after I recovered from BED, I didn't exercise. When I was on the Last Diet Ever I was up before dawn to exercise. And if I could, I'd fit in an exercise class after work at the gym. When the dam broke, the exercising immediately stopped. What was the point? I was defeated.

For the past five years, I've been working on telling myself the truth about exercising. If I want my body to work well, I need it to be strong. This has nothing to do with losing weight. *Exercising has nothing to do with losing weight*, a new belief I'm trying to embrace.

I am working on pulling exercise and food apart. I am successful, sometimes. It's psychologically hard. Sometimes I will intentionally eat "bad" foods after I exercise to demonstrate to myself that I'm not exercising to lose weight. This has been semi-successful. I think I will be able to embrace and fully believe that exercising is something for the health of my body (nice to be able to go up a flight of stairs) and doesn't have to involve restricting. Maybe it can become for me what it should be: a necessary activity people should do regularly for the physical and mental health of their bodies.

I have hope I will continue to work on this aspect of my health. The more I tell myself the truth – exercise for basic health - the more I really begin to believe it. Honestly, I do think I am too easy on myself when it comes to exercising. First of all, I don't really like it. I don't like to get sweaty. I don't get an energy boost from exercising. If anything, it makes me tired.

There are aspects I enjoy about walking. I like looking at nature, being outside, listening to music. Walking also frees my mind to solve problems. I'm a young adult author. It is through walks that I've solved many a character's problem or come up with an exciting plot development.

Given all I like about walking, why don't I do it more? Maybe exercising is more entangled with food restriction than I realize. Maybe I'm lazy. Maybe both.

Luckily, I am a work in progress – and so are you! What I am right now is not the whole story. Where you are right now is not complete. We are people in progress. Today is our story up to this point. There is still the rest of the day and all the tomorrows we have.

Questions to consider:
- What is your relationship with exercising?
- Has it changed over the years?
- Do you enjoy exercising?
- Do you think exercising is important?
- Are exercising and dieting connected in an unhealthy way for you? If they are, is this a relationship you see possibly changing?

Chapter 9: The Devil's Scale

When is a tool not simply a tool? When it is used illicitly.

For me, the scale has never been an objective instrument to measure my weight. Never.

The scale has been the gateway, the gamemaster. I had to please the scale and give her what she wanted to pass through to the dream: normal weight.

There has never been anyone in my life who has had the power over me and my mood like the bathroom scale. The bathroom scale held all the power. This is where the truth would out. This is where all the world could see I was "good" that week (or day before). The scale told me if I ate too much or too little. The scale told me if I was good or bad. Successful or unsuccessful.

She was full of surprises. Usually terrible surprises, but surprises that nonetheless kept me coming back for more. If I tried hard enough, the scale would reward me, right? And the scale was always right. Always told the cold-harsh truth of the matter – I wasn't as good as I thought I was. I should redouble my efforts and eat less, exercise more. *I don't deserve to eat.*

If the scale gave me bad news, it was my fault. Yet another failure.

In the beginning of a diet, I had to muster up the courage to stand on her to see and assess the damage. I could face this horrid scale number because it would be going away, never to be seen again.

The first weeks of a diet, the scale was my friend. She encouraged me, while not letting me get a big head. I would always think my efforts merited more of a loss. But any loss, any negative was welcomed. Kind of.

If the scale was -3 for any given week, that was good. Not great, because great was reserved for -5 or more. I maybe did 'great' once or twice in twenty-five plus years.

A loss of 2 pounds was fine. Average. But was I really average? Certainly, I could do better.

-1.5. Still acceptable, but I could definitely improve.

-1. Okay. Still a loss, but nothing to be proud of. I should stew on this for a while and feel awful for the bad choices I've been making.

-0.5. I mean, give me a break. All that work for a measly half a pound loss? You are a loser. What is wrong with you?

0. Here I'd start to sweat. Definitely not good. Very bad. I must be deceiving myself. Too much peanut butter, not enough water. *You are a disappointment. You will never do it. You should be ashamed of yourself. You will always be fat.*

Anything in the plus meant I should berate myself as an obvious failure. Weight loss isn't rocket science. It's very, very easy. Stop eating. *You don't deserve to eat. Your punishment is to feel demoralized and awful about yourself. All day. You should consider stopping this worthless endeavor, since you obviously are deceiving yourself as to what you are eating. You can't even count calories right. Worthless. Stupid. You don't deserve to be rid of the fat. You deserve your own jail cell of fat. Forever imprisoned.*

There was no winning. I knew this before I stepped on the scale. It had always been the case that both the scale and I knew it had the power to make or break me. It alone could tell me I was good, on the right path. There was no other metric as immediate or visceral as her glowing numbers, just ready to commend or condemn me at a moment's notice.

Countless times I argued with myself about stepping on her. I knew she'd tell me I was trash. But hope is powerful. Maybe, just maybe, I weighed less than the time before. Maybe, by some magic, I was skinnier now than yesterday in which I had gained weight.

When I decided to never go on a diet again, I decided the scale was off limits too. Just as nothing good comes of another round of restricting, getting on the scale is a recipe for disaster.

When I began to recover from BED, I somehow found the courage to stand up for myself at the doctor's office. After calling my name from the waiting room, I was escorted to the scale, per usual. Nervously, I told the nurse I don't weigh because I've got an eating disorder.

I could tell I caught the nurse off guard, but she quickly righted herself and showed me the exam room. I couldn't believe it! Just like that, telling someone what I needed worked. The next time I was at the doctor's office, I worked up my resolve to do the same. It worked again. No one made me weigh. Time and time again, I'd say, "I don't weigh," and they wouldn't weigh me.

When I needed to be weighed for insurance or some other reason, I'd close my eyes. The nurse weighing me would take the information and zero out the scale before I opened my eyes. Something so small, that act of grace, filled me with gratitude. Every nurse at my regular doctor and at the OB/GYN's office treated me kindly. Not one of them made me feel weird about not weighing.

From the time I went into recovery from BED to the moment I embarked on the new path of weight loss medicine[17], I did not weigh myself. I assumed I weighed about 190. This was fine. I could tell my weight wasn't fluctuating more than ten pounds either way because my clothes fit.

For a good eight years I just ate what I wanted and didn't give a thought to the number on the scale. In fact, when I

---

[17] I've been on three different weight loss medicines. I've decided to exclude the names of these prescribed medications because 1) I am not a physician and 2) I think the best medicine for you to take, if you take one, is decided in a conversation between you and your healthcare provider. I've come to think of the medicine as helping me manage my food addiction, much like someone who takes an antidepressant to manage depression.

decided to weigh myself at home a few months into taking the first weight loss medicine I went on, I wasn't sure if we still owned a scale.

I was pleased to be out of the 190s, but the old feeling rushed right back. My self-worth and mood would be tied to the number on the scale if I listened to it. Now on my third weight loss medicine, I think I have weighed myself four times.

I am not mentally healthy enough to use a scale. Even when I see lower numbers my immediate thoughts are, *why isn't this number lower? What is wrong with me? You've been deceiving yourself about your body. You really shouldn't be eating.*

The fact of the matter is I'm not willing to trash talk and berate myself over what the scale says. I do know how my body is doing. I can feel how my clothes fit and how it feels to move around. I don't need a scale to tell me anything about myself.

While I believe this intellectually, I'm conflicted. I'd be lying if I said that I don't care what the scale says about me. I still want her to accept me. Tell me I'm good. I am just no longer desperate for her affirmation. But I see her out of the corner of my eye. She's a wicked mistress and happy to have me under her grasp again.

I can imagine someone without a food addiction reasonably saying, "This seems foolish. If you don't weigh yourself, how can you know if you're out of control? Weight and obesity are not something to play fast and loose with. It's important to know how much you weigh, so you can take appropriate measures. And, as we know, knowledge is power."

No. I say real self-power comes in knowing your body and paying attention to it. I know when my clothes are loose or snug. I know when a double chin appears in a picture and when it recedes. I don't need a scale to tell me the size of my body. And I certainly don't need the mental weight of carrying it around – just another thing to tell me I'm bad.

But I'm not bad. I have a body. My body is the size it is for many reasons. I am not overweight because I am a failure. I am overweight because I have a mental/physical illness.

When I get on the scale, I forget what's really going on with me and I reduce myself to an object. I become the number on the scale. The number is too high, therefore I am no good. It's my fault and I should now berate myself and stew over the number.

Late into the winter during Covid, I weighed myself. I'd been on weight loss medicine for a while and knew I'd lost some weight. In my mind the fantasy bloomed. Maybe I'd be 160 pounds! Maybe … dare I dream it … I'd be in the 150s. I was 169.7.

Fine.

Fine?!? This is awesome! If I never moved from this weight, that would be great. And I know this, but the allure of a small number on the scale is too strong. It has the power to fixate me. Make me feel terrible.

This goes to one of the main points in this book. I have a condition that needs to be managed. I trip up when I think I am no longer a food addict. Even if I'm not actively restricting, binging, or purging, I have the mind of a food addict. The scale is not, and will probably never be, just a scale. It still has the power of a mood-altering drug over me. In my continuing process to manage my condition, the scale is out.

I began this new freer phase of my life with two rules: no diets and no weighing. While I haven't dieted, I have weighed myself since I started taking weight loss medicine.

It's good to reassess personal rules to see if they are still fitting. As I reassess, I see clearly I don't need the scale and I don't want to be held hostage to its numbers. I reaffirm my simple rules: no dieting and no weighing.

Questions to consider:

- What is your relationship to the scale?
- When do you weigh yourself?
- What are your weighing rituals (clothes on or off? Morning?)
- How often do you weigh yourself? Do you think this level of monitoring your weight is helping you?
- What do you think would happen if you didn't weigh yourself for one year? What do you think would happen if you didn't weigh yourself for five years?

Chapter 10: Using Medicine. I'm Not a Cheater.

What I've come to believe is that I have a physical disorder. I've overcome BED, but I will forever be a recovering food addict. My food addiction is a mental disorder that I've learned to make peace with and treat with the respect it deserves.

What does this mean? It means:

- I can't play around with food.
- I don't get to try fad diets.
- I don't entertain ANY form of food restriction for the purposes of losing weight.
- I recognize I've found a balance with my disorder; it hasn't gone away.
- It's a condition that must be managed.

Recovery from my food addiction is more similar to being a recovering alcoholic than being a cancer patient in remission. It's not as if I broke my arm and now it's mended, only to see the break with an X-ray.

No, I'm a food addict. I am fortunately in recovery. The only way to stay recovered is to deal with the problems as they present themselves. To manage it. If I pretend the food addiction is not there, if I refuse to acknowledge it, it's to my detriment.

Continuing to see myself in a process of recovery, a few years ago when I began to gain weight, I was at a total loss. I was on my no dieting ever plan and hadn't restricted for nearly eight years. I wasn't food crazy and I hadn't gained weight – which I gauged by the way my clothes fit, since I refused to weigh myself.

I felt the best I had ever felt about my body and my relationship with food. I loved the arrangement I had come to with food (I could eat what I wanted when I wanted it[18]) and I'd fully embraced my body and weight I'd be for the rest of my life (around 190). So, when I began to gain weight, I was terrified.

I was terrified because I couldn't see a path forward. I knew food restriction was off the table. The only real solution I could see was a bigger body. I am 5'1". I knew I was over 190 pounds. How much more weight could I really handle?

My lack of restricting was working for me. I hadn't gained weight. Not really. I was at a stable weight for a long time and happy with it. I mean that.

If you are a thin person or of normal weight, it might be hard to imagine someone being happy with a BMI that puts them 10 points in the obese category. But I was. I liked my body. I dressed it and treated it well. But the greatest part of the peace I'd made with food was what was going on in my mind.

Crickets.

No food noise. No obsessing about what to eat, when to eat, how much/little to eat. Nothing. My attention was not on my food at all. I just ate what I wanted and went about my merry way.

One reason I was fine with this arrangement – being obese but having a free mind – was that I felt my body had reached a kind of natural weight set point. For at least 20 years, 190 pounds thereabouts was my default setting. I'd start there – or a little higher – lose weight and then gain it back. I would reset at around 190. (If I'm being honest, I think 190 is the

---

[18] A reader of mine said wisely, "Merry, no one can eat what they want whenever they want." Yes, this is true. And yet, my path to freedom has been through embracing this belief. For me, it is through this unmitigated form of freedom that I've overcome the compulsion to binge. The paradox.

comfortable weight number my brain likes. In actuality the weight number was probably slightly higher).

I have no idea how much I'd gained when I decided to mention something to my OB/GYN nurse practitioner. She knew of my weight issues and suggested taking a new weight loss medicine.

While I had considered gastric bypass surgery, I didn't consider myself heavy enough for it. Besides, a friend of mine had the bypass surgery and the half-year of food restriction prep ahead of the surgery was a no-go for me. Shrinking the size of my stomach wouldn't change the mental issues I have with food. I had no doubt I'd figure out how to regrow the size of my stomach to hold all the food I'd be consuming if I started down the path of restriction again.

What I never considered was medicine. I grew up in the 80s. I was horrified with the stories of girls taking pills with tapeworms, afterschool specials of girls on diet speed drugs, and the all-around deleterious effects of illicit weight loss drugs. I surmised they were dangerous and ultimately didn't work anyway. Just another diet and another way to restrict.

But that was then. When I was offered weight loss medicine, I first said no. No way! I wasn't going down this path again! I was out. I was out of the diet game, and I wasn't going to be sucked back in ….

But I was at the upper end of what I thought was an acceptable weight. What felt okay in my own body. What if I did nothing and I gained and gained? While my mind was free of food craziness, if I started to get into the 200s, would my food-addicted mind stay clear?

There were two options: food restrict or not. That's all I saw.

But then, magically, a third way presented itself.

With the weight loss medicine, I was certain I was supposed to food restrict and exercise. The medicine was to help in my diet efforts. What if I took the medicine but didn't change anything else? I could take it and pretend - since I'm a pro at hiding information from myself - that I'm not taking it. No diet, just the medicine.[19]

A new path came into being.

The first months were psychologically difficult. Confronting any food or weight issue is painful and dredges up my all too ready obsessive food monologue. But, after a few months of doing what I resolved to do – take the medicine and not restrict – the mental food noise receded.

I really liked the first drug. Once I settled into it, my relentless food chatter receded into the background. The medicine worked on my brain, telling it I wasn't all that hungry.

The most annoying aspect of that first medicine was getting it filled. It was classified as a controlled substance and there were hoops every month to get it. It also didn't stay in my system long.

Even though it was stressful dealing with getting the medicine, I really liked it. Imagine my surprise when I went to get my monthly supply to find it had been discontinued! That was really upsetting.

I wasn't giving up. I'd been on the medicine for about 9 months and lost the unknown added weight and a bit more. If I had to guess, I was probably between 180 – 185 pounds. I felt good in my body and the food issues were very manageable

---

[19] Thinking back, trying to remember precisely why I decided to try the medicine route is murky in my mind. I suppose I decided to try because I trusted my healthcare provider, who I had a good relationship with. I was curious, but more importantly I was at a crossroads. Dieting was absolutely off the table, but I really didn't want to continue to gain weight. I reasoned, maybe weight loss medicine had come a long way since the 1980s.

since I wasn't restricting. The biggest mental blow back was from the accusing thoughts of how I was "wasting" this opportunity to lose weight. *Imagine what you'd lose if you went on a diet and took the drug!* This thought came often, but I saw it for the trap it was. It was inviting me back into the pit of despair, but I was not tempted. I am 100% convinced that dieting, for me, given my addictions, is nothing more than giving into a disease that only takes and destroys the quality of my life.

Facing the fact that I wasn't going to get the manufacturer to make the drug for me, I went back to my NP. She prescribed a different medicine, which was a twice a day pill. This made me uneasy. I can manage to remember a pill once a day, not consistently twice. And then the pandemic hit.

I was now working from home with no normal schedule in sight. I don't know if I ever made it consecutive days taking the medicine twice a day. I stopped taking the pills because I wasn't being consistent and taking it just once a day didn't work. I know this because I was hungry again.

If I'm hungry I eat. That's my rule. I don't restrict.

While not binging, it was pandemic eating. I was worried about the effects of doing nothing during the pandemic. If I was really in a new stage with my aging body that was going to add extra pounds … I didn't want that. I just wanted my regular fat body.

I went back to my NP. She offered a different medicine; one I'd already turned down because it's a daily shot. My immediate reaction was a big fat 'no.' But, the more I thought and read about it, I decided to try it. I hoped it would work much like the first medicine.

As of the writing of this book, I am still on the daily shot. It took a while to get used to, but it no longer bothers me. In fact, injecting the medicine is a visual and physical reminder that I'm a food addict in recovery, daily managing my condition.

For me, the daily shot makes me feel full on a moderate amount of food, so that I can't eat too much. I can't tell you how many times I've cursed the medicine because I wanted to keep on eating but couldn't because I felt sick.

This is strange to me, because I purged all the way through high school and some afterwards. In the throws of BED, I routinely ate when I was full. Full didn't stop me. Full has never stopped me. Sick didn't stop me either.

But this medicine? It feels like I just don't have the energy to overeat.

My guess is that when I'd eat and get sick, I was controlling the overeating and sickness. But this medicine is working behind the scenes and decides for me when I'll be sick to my stomach. What I mean by this is that there is a delayed reaction and relationship of the nausea and eating.

When I'd binge, I'd eat until I couldn't eat anymore. There was a direct and immediate feeling between the food and being sick. With the medicine, I would eat something and then hours later start to feel sick. Months of this has trained me that eating too much is not worth feeling sick later. I can't tell what's going to make me sick. I think the sick feeling comes or doesn't based on when I take the daily shot and what I've eaten over a period of time. It's the unpredictability of the sickness, coupled with being hit with an upset stomach seemingly out of the blue that is training me to just not eat that much. It's annoying and I hate this side effect, but it's a price I'm currently willing to pay.

I still stand on principle that I eat what I want when I want it. The medicine works on my brain, so that I just don't eat as much. Also, it makes it so that I'm just not all that interested in food. I do hear the voices telling me I'm squandering this golden opportunity to really lose weight if I would just restrict! But I know that is a lie and a sure path to crippling mental illness.

The last time I weighed myself before throwing out the bathroom scale, I weighed 170 pounds. If I could stay at this weight for the rest of my life I'd be thrilled. But I know it's temporary. I know the drug is helping me by calming my brain.

How do I feel about that?

I am proud of myself. I am proud that I am taking care of myself.

At peace.

I have a medical condition and I'm treating my malady with medicine.

I am thankful.

I am not cheating. Taking medicine when you are sick is not cheating.

There was an article in the New York Times recently (5/13/2021) about weight loss medicine. I typically don't read the comments, but I wanted to see how people reacted.

I was not surprised.

The comments were pretty much divided between those who have a food addiction and those who don't.

Those who suffer from food addiction were pleading with the non-addicts to see this as a positive development. A help and relief for those who suffer terribly with this addiction.

Those who aren't food addicts predictably bemoaned that our culture "throws pills" at every problem. *These overweight pieces-of-shit need to eat less and exercise. Problem solved.*

To those who are against using medicine to combat obesity, let me say to you: **managing addiction is smart and brave.**

The person who emerges from clinical depression by way of utilizing anti-depressants isn't cheating.

The person who uses a cast to fix a broken bone isn't cheating.

Using medicine to manage an addiction isn't cheating.

I am fundamentally broken when it comes to food. I am taking control and doing something about it. I will use all the tools available to me: breathing exercises, prayer, meditation, talk therapy, and medicine.[20]

I feel no stigma.

I feel free.

I fully intend to treat my food addiction with medicine[21] until I die.

Questions to consider:
- What do you think about using medicine to manage food addiction?
- Why do you have these beliefs about using medicine to manage food addiction?
- Have you ever tried using medicine to manage a food addiction? What was the outcome?
- What do you consider "cheating" when it comes to managing weight?

---

[20] I understand some might think I'm hypocritical to claim I won't ever diet again, yet I'm taking weight loss medicine. Or maybe the hypocrisy comes with me saying "I'm free" from BED and dieting, but taking weight loss medicine. On the face of it, I see the confusion. You see, I am not taking the medicine to lose weight. I am taking the medicine to calm the problem in my brain surrounding food. It is not an easy balance to find, but this is what works for me. I embrace both refusing to restrict my diet in order to lose weight and taking weigh loss medicine.

[21] The medicine I'm on would be cost prohibitive if I didn't have good health insurance. This is highly problematic. Using medicine as part of a treatment plan to combat food addiction is reasonable, but is not accessible for so many who either don't have any or minimal health insurance. Obesity is an epidemic. Why would we develop treatments and then not make them available due to cost and/or negative social stigma?

- What do you think of the idea of looking at weight management as a medical, social, and psychological issue rather than a simple lack of will-power?

Chapter 11: Is it Really Possible Not to Diet?

Fine, fine. No restrictive diets to lose weight. These types of diets are bad. This is the current mantra of many in the diet community.

I've even seen the no diet diet.

Is this good? It depends.

Just as there is no one-size-fits-all when it comes to food consumption and our bodies,[22] the reason people are overweight and may or may not benefit from a diet varies widely.

People live with different economic realities. We don't all have access to the same resources. Some can afford private chefs, delivered prepared foods, fancy health food grocery stores, local Walmart, or food banks. For some people, their access to food is the local gas station.

People have different physical issues. Consider allergies, genetic disorders, sicknesses.

People have different psychological needs. In addition to eating disorders, consider religious and moral restrictions.

Not everyone on a diet or who is overweight feels bad about it or has an unhealthy relationship with food. Some people who grew up in the average weight range and as they got older, their metabolism changed but not their eating habits, have often found themselves overweight and needing to rethink (or think for the first time) about what to eat to maintain a healthy weight.

---

[22] Again, I find myself tempted to believe the "person as thing" equation of having a healthy weight as a simple matter of energy conversion. Take in X number of calories until you reach healthy weight and then eat X number of calories. Simple.

No, not simple. We are not objects, but subjects; we are persons. We are complicated. To reduce a serious personal issue and the person with the issue to an object is both offensive and ineffectual. Stop it.

While I haven't tried Noom, for obvious reasons, I applaud the approach of attacking the psychological factors that plague some people with weight management issues. I wonder if I had come across something like this when I was a teenager, if I would have avoided my food addiction.

I find the future of weight loss management promising. The food battle is fought and won in the mind, not the mouth. What does or doesn't get eaten have to do with what we tell ourselves, what we need, and how we go about filling those needs.

Realizing some people are addicted to food in a very similar way someone is addicted to drugs or alcohol might shift the conversation away from counting calories to addressing mental health issues. Addressing the addiction. An addiction that must be faced. One that must be named and dealt with.

For decades, I tried everything I could to hide my addiction from myself. I was so ashamed. Countless times I've fantasized about never eating again. If I didn't have to eat, I wouldn't have to make food choices. I wouldn't be caught off guard with a trigger food memory as I ate something, sending me headlong into the rabbit hole of food consuming.

When I was on my Last Diet Ever, I dreamt of swimming in a sea of M&Ms. The feel of the cool, smooth, silky, candy coated chocolate surrounded my body as I pushed through it. I awoke feeling like I'd had a taste of heaven. Heaven was being free of the incessant mental food battle, freed to be surrounded with what I loved and longed for.

On my Last Diet Ever, I cursed food. I hated it as much as I hated my body. Why couldn't I just give it up?

What if I wired my mouth shut? – not practical, I decided.

What if I just drank, something like SlimFast? Tried that. My throat eventually wouldn't let me swallow it. While I like SlimFast, there is only so much I could physically tolerate without getting sick.

There were the months I fantasized about being hospitalized. If I could get admitted to a hospital, they'd take over my eating and I could get a break.

I am broken when it comes to food. I am an addict. That's my reality. So, back to the question. Are all diets bad?

If we understand diets extraordinarily broadly as any food restriction for a time for any reason, then I'd say there is a time and place for diets, even for me.

I can imagine restricting food to get ready for a surgery. I can imagine a time when I might be able to participate in fast days that are part of my religion.

What I say no to is dieting to lose weight. It's not worth it.

I can hear the naysayers in my ear. They say, "Oh, so, you're willing to put yourself at risk for developing hypertension, Type 2 diabetes, heart disease, etc.?"

"Oh, yes, that's what I want!" I respond, sarcastically. Give me a break.

"Well, it's within your power. If you just exercised a little self-control, then you could pull yourself together! Don't you want to live to see your grandchildren? Don't you know excess weight can cut your life short?"

"Oh, thank you very much. I didn't know. Thanks for the heavy dose of shame and fresh despair. I'll just go ahead and add that to my daily floggings. Does that work for you?"[23]

---

[23] I realize not everyone has the same health needs, concerns, and conditions. It might be "easy" for me to recommend eating whatever you want because I don't have a health condition that prohibits me from eating certain foods. If you are dealing with IBS, diabetes, or a nut allergy, eating whatever your heart desires is **terrible advice**. My advice is not one-size-fits-all because people are different, with unique histories and needs. My overarching message in this book for food addicts is, there is hope for you! It may not be traditional, but it is out there. It starts with treating yourself with love and care.

"Okay, if you won't diet for your health or your children, do you know that fat people are discriminated against? They make less money than and are regularly passed over for job promotions compared to their thinner work counter parts."

Oh. My. Word. If you are not keenly aware of the daily discrimination overweight people face … I don't know what to tell you. There's also the issue of getting around in a society that isn't designed for your body.

There's nothing like the fear of breaking someone's chair because of your weight. Nothing like the worry the person sitting in the plane seat next to you will voice their disgust because your hips have spread out of your seat and are touching theirs. Nothing like finding zilch in your size at a shop.

Society is now designed in such a way that healthy foods are more expensive and harder to find.

Society is now designed to require little to no physical effort to get about.

Society is now designed to bombard you with photoshopped images of what our bodies are supposed to look like. Advertisers spend astronomical amounts of money to make us feel bad about our bodies, so we will buy their product and feel better. The United States spends trillions in the beauty and fashion industry, more than the GDP of most other nations.

What is a diet? A diet is a temporary form of restriction until the goal is reached and the restriction ends. Right?

Diets are out. I am canceling them. They are mean, nasty, and false.

What can the obese do instead? Manage their condition and make peace with food. This is not a diet.

No more diets. That's what I declare.

Imagine a culture that gives up on diets and opts for actual mental and physical health. Let's do that instead.

Chapter 12: Living as Obese in a Thin-Obsessed Culture

As a young person, I internalized the images found in the magazines and on TV. The only path to happiness was to look attractive. I needed a thin body like the super models to be good enough.

We all have formative memories. I vividly remember an experience I had in high school with one of my best friends. We were hanging out at the local mall, the Valley Plaza, and in a shop that sold a variety of items. Passing by a rack of calendars, he pointed to a model on a swimsuit calendar and said to me, "You could look pretty like that if you lost weight." He walked on to look at something else, while I felt like I'd been slapped in the face and publicly shamed.

I remember feeling like a deer in headlights. I think he was trying to pay me a compliment. He was saying I was pretty – or at least could be if I lost weight. By this time in high school, I was already dieting and purging regularly. I'm pretty sure I purged my weight in food. If you are bulimic, I am very sorry. I know how addictive that behavior is. I see you. Peace to you.

I purged out of despair. I couldn't stop eating in high school, so the only way out was throwing it up. I was aware of the deleterious effect of purging and that helped me regulate the throwing up somewhat. I didn't want the stomach acid to rot my teeth. I didn't want my heart to stop. I didn't want the purging to show on my fingers.

I didn't want my sickness to show partly (or mostly) because it would mean loss of control. If people knew, really knew, what I was up to, they'd have to put a stop to it. But then I wouldn't be in control anymore.

That's so messed up.

Writing this book is hard. I can't believe all the sick things I've done to my body, all to have a thin, acceptable body. All to be beautiful and loved.

What an impoverished view of beauty and love.

What is beauty?

In this "Spanx" culture, we are to look to Instagram for the answer. We look to Fashion Week, TV, movies, and rock stars. We look to the type of clothes sold in stores, and who they are made for. We watch countless YouTube videos on make-up application. There are clues everywhere as to what is and isn't acceptable.

We look to materialism – conspicuous consumption. Just have more. Money will make you pretty if you don't have natural good looks. Money can buy you a new face and sculpt you a new body. And, by the way, add some fake eyelashes to that face. And thicker brows – while you're at it, why don't you tattoo those brows on. But only temporarily, so you can come back in six months to spend more money as you undergo the needle.

I have made a conscious decision to live as obese in a thin-obsessed world. The reason is not because I don't know about the hazards of lugging around extra weight.

I have made this informed decision because I am aware of the alternatives for me. I can choose to have a healthy mind and a big body or an obsessed diseased mind and an almost normal looking body.

I am my worst critic when it comes to my weight. There is NOTHING a person can say to me or think about me that I haven't tortured myself with.

When I think about dieting, the best way to describe the aversion I have to dieting is by comparing it to a person who has repeatedly burned her hand on a hot stove. You know – intimately know - if you touch that hot stove again you will burn your hand. You have the scarred hand to prove it. The thought of touching a hot stove makes your scarred hand throb and you start to flush, like ants crawling right beneath the skin.

Touch a hot stove? Hell to the no. No way. No thank you.

I don't care what promises are on the other side of the diet, I firmly believe them to be false. Even if I achieve the desired weight, it won't be sustained. And even if it was, *this time*, even if I were successful, at what cost? What psychological torment would I have to endure to get there?

The so-called prize is not worth the price. **I know this deep within myself**. It doesn't seem fair to have to choose between mental or physical health, but as we are all keenly aware, life isn't fair. For me, I have finally chosen mental health.

Mental health looks good on me. It is sooooo lovely to breathe. The freedom I feel, the joy to not have to be on a diet (or about to go on a diet or just failing a diet). My next diet is not starting in the morning or when I get back from vacation because I'm freeeeeeeeeeeee! I never have to diet again. Yay me!

I will never diet again. I have reconciled with being obese. I don't want to be obese, but I finally prize my mental health more. I think this is the best choice.

Honestly, I am threading the needle by taking a weight loss medicine. But the decision I have made is to treat my food issues as to what they are: a sickness. Some illnesses can be treated with medicine.

I would be lying if I said taking weight loss medicine was an easy decision. I thought a lot about jumping back into the fray of giving food a second thought. After eight glorious years of freedom, why would I contemplate going back to prison?

I am in a different place. BED is behind me. Bulimia is in my rear-view mirror. I have an addictive personality. I obsess about some things. When my attention is on food, I obsess about it. Given what I know in my bones – no restrictive eating for weight loss ever again – I am able to move on to the next chapter in my journey of managing my eating addiction.

Chapter 13: Binge Eating Disorder and Long-Term Emotional Consequences

Though I am in recovery from BED, the emotional effects and traumatic memories are still with me.

Sometimes, when I think about the time I spent living with binge eating disorder, I cry. I cry for the woman who experienced that pain. I cry for her extreme distress.

Seemingly out of the blue, some facet of that time will drift through my mind and stop me cold. I want to go to her, hold her, help her to let go of the pain. I want to take it from her.

But I can't.

And you can't take the pain from someone else or yourself.

Pain must be lived and respected.

What I see now, what freed me was not what I thought. I thought my last diet to end all diets freed me from my food addiction.

It didn't because I am a food addict. That is not going away.

But the pain of BED burned out of me – burned out with a white-hot melting fire – the belief that dieting, aka restricting, was acceptable.

It is not acceptable for me anymore than it is acceptable for a drunk to have a drink.

Whenever I stray from my resolution to never restrict, the traumatic memories surface and nips those destructive thoughts.

I know, in my bones, that restriction is the path to my destruction. If you are not a food addict, this surely seems like hyperbole. Right?

But it's not about the food. It never has been. It's about control and biology. When I'm on a diet, the voices are shouting at me from the time I wake up until I am back asleep.

What are you going to eat today? How much is a serving? Don't eat that! You don't deserve to eat. What have you eaten so far? What did you eat yesterday? How much water have you had? No, it was more. When are you going to eat? How long can you wait? You shouldn't wait too long. You should eat now. Don't eat now. You don't deserve to eat. What are you going to eat? What is in the house? How many calories does that have?

This is a real conversation I had with myself many times:

Was that really just a tablespoon of peanut butter or was it a heaping tablespoon of peanut butter? No, it was just a tablespoon. Come, on. You're fooling yourself! It was heaping. Fine, let's measure it. But what about all that's left in the measuring spoon if you measure it? How do I count that? You shouldn't eat peanut butter. Why did you have two scoops of peanut butter? You are so fat! You will always be fat! You are disgusting. No more food for you today. How could you have eaten two scoops? Are you happy with yourself? You will never change. It's the same crap all the time. You promise to change, but you're not changed. You had two scoops. How can you live with yourself? You better spend more time exercising. No more food for you. This played on a loop in my brain for the rest of the day, waking up the next day to regrets of too much peanut butter consumption.

Do you have any idea how much I've berated myself over eating peanut butter?

When I finally gave in and stopped restricting on the Last Diet Ever, the stream of mental beratement didn't stop. It was the same mean, awful talk as I tried to find my way back to the diet. What I thought was sanity.

The sanity I thought I was looking for was when I was riding high on my no-sugar weight loss battle that I thought I won. I wanted back. *Please let me back in!* I pleaded as I ate my way through a cake in the Walmart parking lot. *Please let me be in tight control again! I promise I can do it this time.*

But that was a lie. That was a war I was going to lose. I will always lose if the game is restricting.

The only way to win was to let go. I let go of my heart's desire to be normal weight (which had already shifted from being thin).

I let go of it.

I now see the pain of the BED, the pain of the crushing disappointment, brought me to acceptance.

I accept I cannot diet.

I accept this means I will not have the dream body of normal weight.

Even though I have let go of the diet game, and am through BED, I am still sick. I am still the addict with my addict's past. The pain of what I've suffered still causes me pain.

When someone tells me about their new diet, when someone shows off their weight loss (down 7.5 pounds! Lost 22 pounds for good! Down four pant sizes!), sometimes it draws me right back into the emotional dumpster fire of dieting.

I lived 30 years on a diet. I know the cycle. I know the resolve.

The diet cycle:

Step 1: Unbridled optimism

This time it's going to be different! Those other times are in the past, but this time, I can feel it, *I know it*, it will be different!

Step 2: Living the dream: eating right, exercising, drinking water, telling everyone of your exciting new life!

Step 3: The shine begins to wear off, but you are in it for the long haul.

Step 4: Chinks in the armor: not as fastidious in counting calories, not as much water (I hate peeing all the time), missed workouts.

Step 5: It's over. Shoot. I really thought I'd changed. Oh well, it was not to be.

My diet cycle usually ranged from a day to three months. Very rarely longer.

When I see someone in the cycle, my mind goes into overdrive. I wish them well. I want them to succeed. I remind myself they are not me. I don't know if this is just a diet or if they are a food addict. I want to counsel them to stop it. I want to keep my mouth shut. I know the statistics, which are heavily stacked against them. They will probably yo-yo diet. But hope springs eternal! And that is a good thing. Maybe this time will be different for them.

I now wonder if hope is such a good thing. Is it reasonable to hope to win the lottery? Well, someone is going to win, so why not me?

This kind of hope, for the food addict, when the only tool she is relying on to "win" is self-control is destructive.

The battle scars are real, from the physical stress the body endures from losing and gaining weight, to the emotional baggage.

I am still suffering with the emotional baggage. Mercifully, the scars are healing. The pain isn't as raw from the damage I've inflicted upon myself and the disappointment, but it is still there.

Not treating food addiction as real and demanding people diet – even though we know it's probably a losing gamble - is ludicrous at this late date.

Obesity is an epidemic.[24] It is late in the game to be naive about the complexity surrounding its causes and treatments. We need to do better. This is not a game.

---

[24] Obesity rates have just about tripled in the U.S. in that last 50 years! https://usafacts.org/articles/obesity-rate-nearly-triples-united-states-over-last-50-years/. But this is not a problem for the U.S. only. According to the World Health Organization, obesity rates worldwide have tripled since 1975. https://www.who.int/news-room/fact-sheets/detail/obesity-

Chapter 14: Society, Do Better

The tired and outdated "wisdom" of eat less to deal with the obesity epidemic should sound absurd to our ears. Since we know diets usually fail, should we really treat our mental and physical health like winning the lottery? Rather, what about helping people – early on – to spot food addiction and behaviors that might end in food addiction. Let's educate people on healthy attitudes towards food. While we're at it, maybe we could stop fat shaming. Maybe we could tell people their worth is not dependent on what their body looks like. Maybe we could stop discrimination based on size.

Am I asking to live in a utopia? Probably.

We will not stop fat shaming if money can be made. And I mean lots of money. Who benefits from telling fat people they are gross and should change to be accepted? Society certainly doesn't benefit, if we understand benefiting to be flourishing. Instead, we have a sick society from top to bottom. We constantly hear:

- Of course, it's not just body size (too big or too small).
- Your eyebrows are too thick (or too thin).
- Your hair is to bushy (or too flat).
- Your butt is too big (or too small).
- Your teeth are the wrong color or crooked.
- Your eyelashes aren't full enough.
- Your skin is too uneven.
- Your skin is too dark (or too light).
- Your car is too old.
- Your jeans are last year.

------

and-overweight. The consequences of this epidemic are vast, from the immense burden on our healthcare system, to narrowing possible candidates for the armed forces.
https://www.cdc.gov/physicalactivity/downloads/unfit-to-serve.pdf

- You're too short – wear heels (or too tall – hunch over).
- Your voice is too high (or too low).
- You don't smile (or you smile too much – stop it).
- You don't speak up (or you talk too much).
- You're not confident (or you're too bossy).
- You don't conform enough (or you're sooooo basic).
- You're too introverted – get out more (or you're too extraverted – go home).

OH. MY. WORD! One might conclude that there is nothing right with us! We lack the wrong model/brand of phone. We lack the right clothes, right vacations, right background … right everything. I haven't even addressed what society tells people missing a limb, a sense, or are neuro atypical.

Online, no human body is good enough. Everything needs a filter. We are far removed from reality.

No wonder plastic surgery, debt, depression, loneliness, and suicide are at all-time highs.

Modern day marketing is, for the most part, built on the idea of the following:

- Tell them there is something wrong with them.
- Make them feel like shit because X is wrong with them.
- Act as savior because, guess what, we have the product or service that can fix them!

But we are never fixed. Filling our desire for deep communion with one another will not be met through consumerism. It will not be met from consuming copious amounts of M&Ms, new clothes, alcohol, pills … pick your poison.

Consumerism is poison because it diverts and distracts our attention from what brings lasting human happiness.

The message I received early on from our image obsessed culture was: have the right body and you will be loved and have a good life.

No one ever said this to me because it's absurd! No one could say this with a straight face for it's clearly false.

But years in line at the checkout counter told me: beautiful bodies are thin. Decades of watching film and TV. The only stories worthy of being told were of people with good (aka thin) bodies. The only people deserving of love and attention were those with thin bodies.

No one had to tell me. I got it. Thin = acceptance = good life.

Why have I brought all of this up in a book about BED recovery? When people say, "It's simple. Just watch what you eat and make healthy choices," I look at them like they're aliens.

It's not about the food. It's about the person's internal narrative. What are they telling themselves and why?

I have breathed the air of thin bodies as the only ones that are beautiful my entire life. I believe we gravitate towards the beautiful. We all want to be seen and cherished and loved.

I, little ol' me, am supposed to look at all this societal programming and call bullshit?

Well, now I can, even though I'm still in its snare.

We are asking 12-year-olds to call bullshit? I call bullshit on your bullshit. There is no f#*@ing way I am going to blame myself for years of messed-up ideas of beauty and acceptable bodies because I wasn't mature enough to internalize the truth of the matter. There is no way a teenager is at fault for being unable to see through the bullshit of trillions of dollars of marketing and trickery aimed at them to make them feel inadequate.

Chapter 15: Fat Shaming

I learned to fat shame in Jr. High.[25] Once I began to care what I looked like, what clothes I wore, and what my body was supposed to be, I quickly internalized the relentless message from my society: thin is good. Thin bodies are the best. Fat bodies are gross. Thin bodies are deserving. Fat bodies should not be seen. Avert your eyes.

The message was more encompassing than just being thin – I was also being fed the message that youth was better than age (wrinkles? Gray hair? Never!). Money was terribly important. Consuming is what you were born to do. You need other people's approval to be able to approve of yourself. The "lessons" go on and on.

I learned to unconsciously size up the room as to where I was in the pecking order of goodness, determined by where I stood in terms of heaviness. Many times, much of the time, I was the fattest person in the room. Shoot.

Even as a teenager I knew this was messed up, but I couldn't help it. I looked at the thin people and thought they had it easy. Their bodies were good. Even though I knew the people in those bodies had problems, they were thin people problems.

What would it be like to have a thin body? How would it feel to wear shorts with ease? To not have perpetually burning chaffed thighs in the summer? What if my underwear didn't constantly ride up? What would it feel like to walk around without embarrassment?

Everyone had problems, but everyone could see mine. I felt exposed. Constantly judged. Now I see I was the only one obsessed with my weight. The only one who constantly shamed me was me. But I didn't know that as a teenager.

---

[25] I'm letting you into my private thoughts and world. I am 100% against fat shaming and would "cancel" my own thoughts if I could.

As a teenager I dealt with poor self-esteem, depression, bulimia, and countless failed diets, all before I graduated high school. All with a smiling face. I was good at hiding.

When I went to college, I left the depression and bulimia behind - for the most part. I dabbled a bit in college and beyond with throwing up, but it wasn't a sustained or prolonged effort. What I didn't leave behind was the orientation I had towards fat. Fat was bad. I was fat, so I was bad.

When I was sick, I deserved it because I was fat and didn't eat a healthy diet. I deserved to be sick. It was a just punishment or outcome.

When other people were sick, they didn't deserve it. Since they weren't overweight, any sickness *happened* to them. They weren't responsible. I was. Did I, then, assume other fat people who were sick deserved it? No. My obsession was narrow. Me against the skinny people.

When I was younger, I looked at thin bodies with envy. I wanted what they had. What did they have? In my imagination they had:

- The potential to be picked up by their lover.
- They could be carried over the threshold.
- They could be given a piggy-back ride.
- They could be hugged in such a way that their lover's arms wrapped all the way around their bodies.
- They could sit on their lover's lap without fear of crushing them.

The thin could attract a lover. The thin could command a room. Thin was power. A superpower I had no access to.

Now that I've aged and gained a certain amount of perspective, my obsession has receded. I am no longer obsessed with thin bodies, but I've retained a fascination with what it would feel like to have a body freed of excess weight.

As I people watch I imagine what it feels like to be in their bodies. Thin person, what does it feel like to walk down the street? Thin runner, how does it feel to run? As I watch a clip of a thin woman doing yoga, what does it feel like to move your arms like that? Sit in that position without your hips or boobs in the way? I imagine it feels like sunshine. Then I wonder, does it feel like sunshine to her? Does she know what she has, to have a body that follows its design?

When I look at others with less-than-ideal bodies, based on easily accessed societal ideals, I wonder what they think and how it feels to be in their skin. I first hope they are not sick in the head like I am. I wish they don't want another body, that they are free of the constant personal persecution that followed me for twenty-five years. I wonder if their extra weight makes them sad or if they even care at all. I wonder if they are proud of their bodies.

It's when I realize I was sick for so long – twenty-five years! - I feel sorry for myself. I'm a fixer. I like to fix things for people. I wish, deeply, I could have rescued myself from decades of worthless worry and trauma. I dumped so much of my mental energy and life on destructive thoughts and actions. What a waste.

Fat shaming is woven into the fabric of our society. It's in the air we breathe, so much so it seems normal to shame and marginalize those overweight. Every part of society ought to be reflected in art: film, television, books, dance, painting, photography, video games, and so on. We have an unhealthy and unrealistic view of our country and the world at large when what is represented in art is not reflective of the actual community.

Think about the kinds of people you see on television. How many of them are overweight? Over the age of 45? Disabled?

Do you know 76% of Americans are overweight or obese?[26]

Do you know 26% of Americans have some kind of disability?[27]

Do you know 34% of Americans are 45 and older?[28]

There are 60 million Hispanic people in the United States (18%).[29] How many Hispanics are represented in the culture?

There are many ways we can talk about representation and lack of it. We could look at the US and ask if our media accurately reflects the rich diversity of the population.

We know the answer is 'no.' We know what we see in media as "normal" isn't normal at all.[30]

Today there is a body-positive movement. This I whole-heartily applaud. Your worth has nothing – hear me NOTHING – to do with the size of your body. Independent of your size and body, you ought to find clothes to wear, a place to sit comfortably, jobs and job promotions, and a real place in all forms of media. The development in the last few years of the body positive movement seeks to normalize all kinds of bodies. While not new, the body positive message has picked up steam. Unsurprisingly, there is a backlash against it.

Body Positive Message: You are perfect the way you are! Love the skin you're in! You are beautiful! You don't need to change a thing! Embrace your size!

---

[26] https://www.cdc.gov/nchs/fastats/obesity-overweight.htm

[27] https://www.cdc.gov/ncbddd/disabilityandhealth/infographic-disability-impacts-all.html#:~:text=61%20million%20adults%20in%20the,is%20highest%20in%20the%20South.

[28] https://www.census.gov/prod/cen2010/briefs/c2010br-03.pdf

[29] https://www.pewresearch.org/fact-tank/2020/07/07/u-s-hispanic-population-surpassed-60-million-in-2019-but-growth-has-slowed/

[30] Since this book is about food addiction, I am focusing on the lies associated with body images that flood our culture.

Body Positive Backlash: Do you know the statistics associated with being overweight and obese? Do you not know you are at increased risk for X health conditions? Don't you know you are reducing your lifespan as well as putting an enormous burden on the healthcare system and economy? Besides, fat is gross. I don't want to see your fat body. Here, try this diet. All you need is a little willpower. It's hard for me too, but I watch what I eat. So should (and could) you.

What I see in this "discussion" is our increasing inability to make meaningful distinctions. We are all or nothing. We are left or right in politics. We are right or wrong. No gray. No room for the truth.

So, what is the truth? Here are a few:

- Everyone has different experiences with food and body weight and as such, we ought not make the mistake of thinking everyone thinks as we do. Your experience with your body and your weight is your experience.
- Diversity is a good!
- We should recognize the basics of how we work as biological creatures. It does no one a service to pretend there aren't serious health risks associated with being overweight.
- We ought not assume someone who is overweight is unaware of the health risks. If someone overweight is aware of the health risks, then we might seriously consider alternative explanations for why that person is overweight.
- Losing weight and maintaining a healthy weight is not as easy as some assume or make it out to be.
- We should stop assuming all overweight people are unhealthy and normal weight people are healthy. Health is not a one-size-fits-all or discernable from a visual glance.
- We should not assume being overweight has to do with a lack of moral fortitude.

- We all need to seriously reassess how to treat all persons with dignity and respect.

Chapter 16: Personal Responsibility

I am a fierce defender of freedom. Freedom of the freewill variety. I believe that personal, internal freedom, is an essential feature of being a person. Internal freedom is necessary for ethics to work. I must be able to choose to be good or bad. If I can't choose my actions, praise and blame, heaven and hell, are meaningless.

Choice is an essential feature of being a human person. If you disagree with me, you've proven my point.[31]

The conversation of whether we are free or determined is a long philosophical debate well over 2,500 years old. I don't think it will be solved in a book about a very different topic. Nonetheless, personal freedom is relevant for our current discussion.

I am an existentialist of sorts. I believe we are the sum total of our choices. While the world happens to us, we decide what it means. For example, if you get in a car accident, what does it mean? Well, you might say, "Merry, it means my car is totaled!" Fine, sure. What I'm asking is, what does it mean to you? Is this a good thing or a bad thing? Are you happy the car is gone? Sad? Frustrated? Angry? Put-out? Indifferent?

The point is, the car is gone, but what does it mean to you? *You decide* what it means to you.

Your friend stabs you in the back (metaphorically), what does it mean to you? Do you feel compassion for her because she must be really hurting to turn on you? Do you turn around

---

[31] If you think we don't have freewill, then you are not free to think through my position and conclude I am right or wrong. Without free will you are some kind of organic computer spitting out results. Personal internal freedom is an essential feature of being a person – even if some individual person is unable to act in a free manner due to a certain situation (infant, sleeping, medical condition, etc.) The exceptions don't disprove the rule.

and stab her back? Do you try to repair the relationship? Do you drop your friend from all your social media sites and try to get her "canceled?"

It depends. Of course it depends. But what does it depend on? You. Your choices. What are you going to do, how are you going to think about the car and friend situation? It is not a forgone conclusion as to what any situation means. You, the chooser, get to decide.

Are you psychologically free to choose any and every option available to you? I would say, "No." In fact, I think we have limited "live" choices when it comes to deciding what we do next. While it's possible for you to steal a car or rob a bank to replace the smashed car, that's not a real option for most of us.

While we have choices in every situation, those choices are not everything physically possible for us to choose. Our physical restrictions in addition to our psychological limitations play huge roles as to the alternate choices we consider and which we pick.

So, we are the sum total of the choices we make, even if those choices are severely limited by external physical circumstances and internal psychological states.

We have choices over much that takes place in our mind. But sometimes we are limited. Same with our bodies.

For example, let's consider running. We can choose to run or not to run. That is, unless we are in an accident and become a paraplegic, get lung cancer and are too winded to run, develop arthritis in our knees making running too painful. The list goes on.

Let's look at these physical ailments. They may have been caused by something we did (Meg ran a red light because she was on the phone, causing a severe car accident leaving her without the use of her legs; Jasmine smoked a pack of cigarettes for thirty years, contributing to her lung cancer; John developed arthritis because he used to do party tricks in which he popped his knees in and out of their sockets, triggering the arthritis). These aliments might have been caused through no fault of ours (someone ran a red light and the wreck left Meg a paraplegic; Jasmine never smoked or was around secondhand smoke and got lung cancer anyway; John never did knee-popping party tricks, but everyone in his family has arthritis and he got it too. Genetics).

Once the damage is done to our bodies, the main issue in dealing with the situation is not living in the past as to how the damage came about, but how to move forward. This moving forward will include making peace with the past. We are welcome to beat our fists into the wind, angry at the world. But to live this way robs us of living our best lives. I don't recommend it.

We are free beings and therefore responsible for our actions.

Am I responsible, though, for my weight problem and food addiction? Yes and no. Here lies an uncomfortable duality I live with. I am internally free in many respects to act and respond to my environment, but there are some internal responses that are not always under my control. I am responsible to act in a healthy way insofar as I am able. When I am unable, I am not morally responsible for my actions.

Being overweight is as seldom straight forward as many pretend.

Are some people overweight out of sheer willed neglect and lack of moral fortitude? I suppose.

Since we know the overweight are laughed at, constantly shamed, are passed over for jobs and promotions, and at high risk for serious health issues, why are people overweight?

I suppose you could conclude the overweight are entirely responsible for their condition. While you might presume this, it is concluded out of sheer laziness and lack of moral seriousness.

Instead, let's be thoughtful and serious. The next chapter examines factors that contribute to obesity in our culture.

Chapter 17: Extenuating Causes that Contribute to Obesity

We will continue to lose the fight to turn the tide in the obesity epidemic if we insist on pushing the lie that an overweight BMI is due to simple lack of self-control.

If lack of self-control isn't the (only) issue, then what is? The following, while certainly not an exhaustive, list of risk factors for being overweight and/or obese shows us the various issues people face.

Food deserts

A food desert is a place where it is hard to near impossible to get fresh food, notably fruits and vegetables. Food deserts are usually found where there are small and marginalized populations, many abandoned or vacant homes, and where residents who have lower levels of education, lower incomes, and higher rates of unemployment live.[32]

> "Food deserts are also a disproportionate reality for Black communities, according to a 2014 study from Johns Hopkins University. The study compared U.S. census tracts of similar poverty levels and found that, in urban areas, Black communities had the fewest supermarkets, white communities had the most, and multiracial communities fell in the middle of the supermarket count spectrum."[33]

Just because you have a population center, that does not mean there will be a grocery store close enough to get anything but processed foods. 19 million Americans live in food deserts. The food access they have is mostly found in convenience stores, gas stations, liquor stores, and fast-food restaurants. To add insult to injury, buying food at gas stations and convenience stores not only makes for a nutritionally deficient

---

[32] https://www.aecf.org/blog/exploring-americas-food-deserts/
[33] https://www.aecf.org/blog/exploring-americas-food-deserts/

diet, those processed foods are often more expensive. As they say, it's expensive to be poor in America.

Imagine for a moment you are a 25-year-old mother of two. You live right at the poverty line and don't have access to personal or public transportation. What do you think you are going to be eating and feeding your children? You will feed them what you have access to and can afford.

Is it really appropriate to fault people for not eating healthy foods when they lack access to them?

Poverty

According to the USDA, 35.2 million Americans lived in food-insecure households in 2019. People of color in America were roughly more than twice as likely to suffer food insecurity (Black 19.1%, Hispanic 15.6% to their white counterparts 7.9%).[34]

There are those who live near healthy foods but are shut out due to the cost. Take the above mother, making the same income. Even if there are healthy choices, she can spend $2.68 for a 6-ounce bag of fresh spinach that will last one to two meals, or $2.27 for a box of 12 bags of Top Ramen, and the kids like the Ramen and hate the spinach.

Is it really appropriate to fault people for eating only those foods they can reasonably afford?

Upbringing

Kids eat what they are given. If you grow up eating fast food, fried food, a diet lacking in fruits and vegetables and heavy in sugars and processed foods, those are the foods that are normal to you. Those are the foods you gravitate to due to habit that runs further back than conscious memory.

In a 2021 University of Riverside study, eating copious amounts of sugar and fat in childhood, even if the adult

---

[34] https://www.npr.org/2020/09/27/912486921/food-insecurity-in-the-u-s-by-the-numbers

changes her eating habits, has long term negative residual effects.[35]

Is it really appropriate to fault adults for eating the way they were raised to eat?

Coping mechanisms

The world is a rough place. We all find coping mechanisms to help us get through the difficult times. And as we know, difficult times find many of us daily. Wouldn't it be wonderful if we all had healthy ways to deal with adversity? Yes, yes it would.

But this is not the case. As young children we find ways to self-sooth. Some rock themselves, read, play sports, bite their fingernails, take baths, lose themselves in the void of their phones, endless internet and games. Some suffer so horrendously, their personality splits to handle the abuse. Many children turn to the easy comfort of food.

As we age, some find meditation, exercise, and prayer, while others cope through drugs, alcohol, sex, or food.

Many of us employ a variety of ways to deal with our situations, depending on what is physically and psychologically available to us. Coping mechanisms can easily become habits. This is good when the coping mechanisms are healthy and appropriate.

When the coping mechanism is destructive, look out. We find ourselves coping with the harsh world in a way that makes our tough situation worse.

When food is the coping mechanism, addiction is a possible outcome.

Is it really appropriate to fault people for using food as a coping mechanism, a strategy many have used since childhood?

---

[35] https://www.sciencedaily.com/releases/2021/02/210203090458.htm

The expense of healthy foods

Who can afford the healthy foods? Certainly, there are many people who can afford fresh fruits and veggies, clean and not prepackaged foods. No fast-food, but food prepared with health in mind.

Since healthy foods tend to be more expensive, many people do not have the luxury of buying them because the demands on their paychecks are immense: phone bill, mortgage, car(s) payment, electric and gas bill, garbage and sewer bill, streaming services, memberships of all kinds, house insurance, car insurance, life insurance, health insurance, saving for retirement, clothing for everyone in the household, furniture, house upkeep, vacations, entertainment, dry cleaning, kid expenses (from conception until always), and food.

Good and healthy foods feel easier to skimp on because cheap food:

1. Tastes good to many
2. Is faster in this fast-paced world
3. Is easier
4. Is cheaper

My husband wanted to make a steak meal. The two steaks we split between five people cost $21 and some change. In addition to steak, we had baked potatoes and salad. The meal, all in, was around $25. Instead, we could've gone through a drive-thru and eaten off the dollar menu. That would have been cheaper, quicker, easier, taken no planning, cooking, or cleaning afterwards.

Is it really appropriate to fault people for eating cheaply when there are too many demands on the paycheck, a paycheck that hasn't kept up with inflation in decades? Ask yourself if you had to choose, which one of the following would you choose to pay for: access to the internet and a smart device – or a constant diet of fresh food?

Sugar in everything

Guess what? Most of us like sugar. Our brains love sugar. Guess what else? Food manufactures put sugar in almost everything. Three out of four products in the average US grocery store have added sugar.[36]

It is estimated Americans consume 66 pounds of added sugar every year. This is added sugar and doesn't include sugars naturally occurring in food. The total sugar we consume, annually, is close to 150 pounds!

While the USDA does not have a daily sugar limit recommendation, the American Heart Association recommends no more than 9 teaspoons for men, 6 teaspoons for women, and 3 to 6 teaspoons for children. In case you are wondering, the average sugar in a 12-ounce soda is 10 teaspoons of sugar.[37]

We eat too much sugar. Added sugar has no health benefits, is simply extra calories, and addictive. Some claim sugar is as addictive as cocaine.[38]

---

[36] https://www.healthyfoodamerica.org/sugartoolkit_overview This site has tons of cool graphs.

[37] https://www.heart.org/en/healthy-living/healthy-eating/eat-smart/sugar/how-much-sugar-is-too-much; https://sugarscience.ucsf.edu/dispelling-myths-too-much.html#.YIgYwpBKg2w. See https://www.cdc.gov/nutrition/data-statistics/added-sugars.html for a breakdown on sugar consumption by age and race. Here is a nice graphic about sugar in our foods https://cdn.trendhunterstatic.com/phpthumbnails/214/214162/214162_1_600.jpeg, and follow this link for a graphic illustrating the US consumption of sweeteners from 1822-2005. https://d3n8a8pro7vhmx.cloudfront.net/heatlhyfoodamerica/pages/388/attachments/original/1509030949/sweetnerersGraph3.gif?1509030949

[38] https://www.addictioncenter.com/drugs/sugar-addiction/

Is it really appropriate to fault people for consuming inappropriate amounts of sugar (which may be addictive) when it is added to the vast majority of our foods?

Fast-Food

Before I had children, I swore I'd never take them to McDonald's. It's bad for them. And then I had kids. McDonald's is in the landscape of their childhood. They have all gotten stuck in the McDonald's Playplace when they were little.

Why? Why would I have allowed fast-food to be part of their childhood diets? Because I like fast-food. Truth be told, I still like McDonald's. The fries call to me. Even the hamburgers, and I have watched the documentaries that should have scared me away from mass meat consumption.

Fast-food is quick, easy, has food that appeals to everyone in the minivan, and when the children were younger we'd drive to the next town over to spend a morning in the play area.

This is my experience, and I think it is much the same for many Americans. According to the CDC, 84.4 million (36.6%)[39] Americans consume fast-food every day. Why is this problematic? A diet filled with fast-food is a diet filled with excess sugar, salt, fat, and calories.

Is it really appropriate to fault people for regularly consuming fast-food when fast-food is part of the fabric of our society, where on any given day one third of Americans are eating fast-food?

Genetics

According to the Obesity Medicine Association:

> "[R]ecent studies suggest that genetics contribute to 40-70% of obesity with the discovery of more than 50 genes that are strongly associated with obesity. While changes in the environment have significantly

---

[39] https://www.cdc.gov/nchs/products/databriefs/db322.htm

increased obesity rates over the last 20 years, the presence or absence of genetic factors protect us from or predispose us to obesity.

More commonly, people who have obesity have multiple genes that predispose them to gain excess weight. One such gene is the fat mass and obesity-associated gene (FTO), which is found in up to 43% of the population. In the presence of readily accessible food, those with the fat mass and obesity-associated gene may have challenges limiting their caloric intake. The presence of this gene and other genes can cause:

- Increased hunger levels
- Increased caloric intake
- Reduced satiety
- Reduced control overeating
- Increased tendency to be sedentary
- Increased tendency to store body fat."[40]

By no means am I suggesting our genetic makeup is our fate. According to a Harvard medical study, "What's increasingly clear from these early findings is that genetic factors identified so far make only a small contribution to obesity risk-and that our genes are not our destiny: Many people who carry these so-called 'obesity genes' do not become overweight, and healthy lifestyles can counteract these genetic effects."[41]

The point here is to keep in mind that while genes don't have to determine us, it is a disservice to not recognize we are biological creatures with some built-in tendencies, for good or for ill.

---

[40] https://obesitymedicine.org/obesity-and-genetics/
[41] https://www.hsph.harvard.edu/obesity-prevention-source/obesity-causes/genes-and-obesity/

Is it really appropriate to fault people for their genetic make-up, coupled with a society that encourages (rather than discourages) overeating?

Abuse

We know abuse markedly increases the likelihood of developing obesity as an adult.[42]

Children are abused in many horrific ways.[43] According to the National Children's Alliance, 700,000 children are abused in the U.S. every year.[44] Abuse is not limited to our childhood years. One in four women and one in six men are victims of sexual abuse during their lifetime.[45]

Is it really appropriate to fault people for their obesity that is rooted in abuse?

Lack of education

Some people have weight issues due to lack of education. Dr. Alan Schwartzstein reflects on a CDC report about the connection between excess weight and education.

> "The thing that struck me as I read the CDC report was the correlation between education and obesity. As the level of education rises, the rate of obesity drops. Adults who didn't finish high school had the highest level of obesity at 35.5 percent, followed by high school

---

[42] https://www.sciencedaily.com/releases/2014/09/140902092947.htm; https://www.theguardian.com/society/2017/sep/27/obesity-childhood-trauma-sugar-tax; https://www.ajpmonline.org/article/S0749-3797(07)00155-9/abstract

[43] https://americanspcc.org/child-abuse-statistics/

[44] https://www.nationalchildrensalliance.org/media-room/national-statistics-on-child-abuse/

[45] https://centerforfamilyjustice.org/community-education/statistics/

graduates (32.3 percent), those who attended college (31 percent) and college graduates (22.2 percent)."[46]

Is it really appropriate to fault someone for their eating issues when their lack of education is a contributing factor?[47] If you don't know, are you still responsible?

The pace and structure of modern America

When is there time to cook? And why would I choose to cook when it can be more expensive, doesn't always taste better than fast options, involves planning (and therefore rotting food in the refrigerator), and I must do dishes?

With most adults working, who has the time to cook? Who has the time to plan the meals? Who has the time to shop? Who has the time to clean up? Every day? Three times a day?

The fabric of our lives center around food. Every holy day, every holiday, every special occasion – let's eat! Not just eat, but feast!

Meeting friends? Let's eat!

Socializing with your church people? Let's eat!

Birthday? Office cake!

New baby? Let's have a buffet!

Family reunion? BBQ!

Is it really appropriate to fault people for following the norms, customs, and structure of the society they live in?

---

[46] https://www.aafp.org/news/blogs/leadervoices/entry/20171120lv-patiented.html#:~:text=As%20the%20level%20of%20education,college%20graduates%20(22.2%20percent).

[47] If it were just a matter of education, how do we explain that 8% of doctors are obese and 34% are overweight?
https://www.medscape.com/features/slideshow/lifestyle/2014/public/overview#2

Is this just a bunch of excuses?

Blame is easy. It's our primary default false refrain with obesity. It's your fault. You are overweight. Do something about it. End of story.

This is offensive. This is to talk to persons as though they are non-persons. Why is any given person overweight/obese? Each person is a person with a past, present, and future. Each person has a story. You have a story which belongs to you.

Obesity is complex. You are complex. To suggest it is as simple as the detached mechanics of energy in vs. energy out is to mistake people for machines. We are not machines, and this simple mathematics offers a false sense of understanding of the problem. If you don't understand the problem, the REAL solution will remain elusive.

There are many contributing factors, such as food deserts, poverty, upbringing, coping mechanisms, the expense of healthy food, sugar in everything we eat, fast-food, genetics, abuse, lack of education, and fabric of society that contribute to what and why we eat.

What, then, is the solution? We ought to recognize there are some things beyond our personal control and some things within our control. For what is in our control, we can work toward finding healthy solutions. For those factors out of our current control, we may look to see if those issues can be changed, fixed, or removed.

I believe in freedom. Even with the odds of your past, society, and genetics trying to pull you in directions you don't want to go, you are ultimately free.

The freedom I have found is in acceptance. I am a food addict. I don't see that changing. It's when I stopped participating in my 30-year-old battle of fighting my inordinate desire to both consume food and my desire to control everything I put in my mouth, I found my solution in the obesity war; I opted out.

I found a third way.

I discovered my third way by critically analyzing, given the outside and interior factors bearing down on me, what I wanted in life the most. What I needed.

I want to live in peace with my body and mind.

I discovered peace for me was not found in living a restrictive lifestyle.

Peace came with the recognition that I am an addict. My condition needs to be recognized and managed. My mantra (I am not on a diet. I can eat whatever I want) is the balm that calms the food addiction. I am free. And with this freedom I have found, I am now responsible in a way that I wasn't when I was psychologically tied in a million knots when I dealt with bulimia in high school or battled (and won!) binge eating disorder.

I am free to see my condition as complex. I am free to see what ways I am directly responsible for my addiction, and to recognize the causes out of my control. I am freed from being gutted and stuck in disappointment at my 30 years of failure. I am free from the big cultural bully that says I'm fat and gross and it's all my fault, which I could change if I wasn't so morally weak.

I am free from the compulsion to diet until the day I die. I completely and utterly reject that future. I have found a new, freer future. I am incredibly grateful to be free.

I am freed from the lie that says my lack of willpower is the only cause of my food addiction and move forward in truth.

Chapter 18: Moving Forward

How do we change our past? We don't. The past is gone and no longer exists.

Does this mean we must stay hostage to our bad experiences, turmoil, habits, and addictions? No.

What I suggest is reframing your past. Reframing involves taking a situation and looking at it from different points of view.

Think of a painting or photo you have in your bedroom, living room, or office. If the picture has been hanging in your house for years, there's a good chance you barely notice it because it's part of your normal landscape.

The same thing happens to our internal thoughts and dialogues. We tell ourselves stories over and over until they recede into the background, and we don't "see" them anymore. We replay ideas over and over, which is fine if those thoughts are healthy. But when the messages are detrimental, we suffer.

How can we be free from negative and false obsessive thoughts? Change the frame.

Take me, for instance. I had the unrelenting belief that I didn't deserve to eat. Why? Eating leads to fat. Fat is bad. I am fat. Therefore, I don't deserve to eat.

When I looked and really examined this belief, I was able to see it was a false belief, which set me on the path to a new way of thinking and dealing with the false belief whenever it pops up.

How do you reframe a belief? To reframe a belief or memory, treat what you are working on as if you are a detached scientist in a white lab coat. An objective detective.

First, state the thought claim under investigation: I don't deserve to eat.

Secondly, investigate the claim through the asking of a series of questions.

Question 1: What exactly is the belief in question?

The scientist would ask questions for clarification. Certainly, this person doesn't mean they don't deserve to eat sweets or expensive meats, right? The issue certainly isn't about all food?

> Interviewing Self: *So, self, what do you really mean? Do you mean all foods?*
> Self: Yes, even apples. The only food that gets a pass is water and celery. Maybe tomatoes … but not too many tomatoes. Those must be watched as well. Celery must be monitored because eating too much can lead to other food related problems. So, yes, I don't deserve to eat because, as I said, eating leads to fat. Fat is bad. I am fat. Therefore, I don't deserve to eat.

Once the interviewing self has clarification about the claim under investigation, she can move to the next question.

Question 2: Is this belief objectively true? Why or why not?

This is a false belief. I am a person with a biological body. If I don't eat, I die. Eating is a basic human right. It is patently absurd to think I don't deserve to eat.

Question 3: What would I say to someone else who had this belief?

If a friend told me she secretly believes she doesn't deserve to eat, I'd be shocked and sad. How could this wonderful, intelligent woman have such a belief?

My first move would be compassion.

> Interviewing Self: *I'm so sorry you feel this way. You must know this is absurd. Nonetheless that's what you're dealing with, so that's what we are dealing with.*

My second move would be a dose of reality.

Interviewing Self: *Let's suppose you're right. This means you are saying you don't deserve to live. Do you believe this?*

Self: It turns out I think I deserve to live.

Interviewing Self: *So, since you believe you deserve to live, you see how these thoughts are incompatible? Does this belief, that you shouldn't eat, bring you joy or health?*

Self: Turns out it doesn't.

Interviewing Self: *Do you see this thought is false? Do you see it as a lie, objectively?*

Self: Turns out I do see it as a lie and objectively false.

Question 4: Is there another way to think about this idea?

Interviewing Self: *You see this is a false belief, but it still plagues you. Am I getting this right?*

Self: Yes.

Interviewing Self: *Okay, let's see if we can think about this in another way. Since you now see this is a false belief, a belief that has gripped and paralyzed you and doesn't help you, what could you do about this thought?*

(Here you are giving yourself a chance to find the solution that is from the inside instead of imposed from the outside. You are calling on personal agency and creativity.)

Self: Well, when I have that thought, I could talk to it. I could name it as false. Would that work?

Interviewing Self: *Is that something you think you could do? How would you do this?*

Self: I could talk to the thought out loud. I could call the thought a liar to its face.

Interviewing Self: *Would that make the thought go away?*

Self: I don't know. I kind of doubt it. I've had this false belief for so long … so, maybe I don't worry about the thought. Maybe, every time it pops up and accuses me, I tell it the truth. That I do deserve to eat. That it's absurd to think otherwise. Maybe I just commit myself to face and not hide from the idea whenever it comes.

I had the belief that I don't deserve to eat. I had it, but no longer. Am I saying I'm free of this thought? I was free for years, but since I've picked up looking at my weight and dealing with it medically, the same old thoughts came to accuse and assault me.

But this time, I'm not having it. I was able to recognize the thought "you don't deserve to eat" as false. When I have that thought, a thought that's been hanging around for the last couple of days, I call it out. I have a conversation with myself as to why it's false. I tell myself I am not on a diet and can eat what I want. I tell myself to stop it (which I found is a less successful strategy).

What I do is address the false beliefs. My food addiction thrives in darkness. So, I pull it into the light. I have a conversation with those thoughts. Yesterday in the grocery store, I had a full conversation with those thoughts, claiming over and over, out loud, so I could hear myself say that I am not on a diet and can eat what I want. Of course, I deserve to eat. That's the dumbest thing I've ever heard! I am not on a diet and can eat what I want.

The other day while eating dinner with my husband, I told him I was having a hard time with food. I told him about this current bout of food addiction irrational thoughts.

I told him the idea bouncing around in my head was, "You don't deserve to eat."

I'd caught him off guard. I could tell by his reaction, "you don't deserve to eat" is a crazy, false thought.

He said, "I had no idea you thought that way."

And then I realized. I don't think I've ever told anyone that haunting false belief.

Seeing it through his eyes – as bizarre – helps me see it more clearly for what it is: A total and utter falsity.

I return to my defense: I'm not on a diet and can eat what I want. That is my mantra. I say it because it's what I'm committed to. Sometimes I backslide. A tell-tale sign is when the thought of not eating - or holding out as long as I can to eat – pushes into my mind. I combat those false ideas with the truth. The truth never gets old. I never tire of telling myself the truth. Sometimes it's frustrating to deal with the same old crap. But, oh well. I'm no longer taking the backseat and wishing those thoughts away. It's like seeing fleas on a cat, again, and wishing they would jump off and die, taking their eggs with them. But that's not a wise method of cat flea removal. That's the path to a flea infestation.

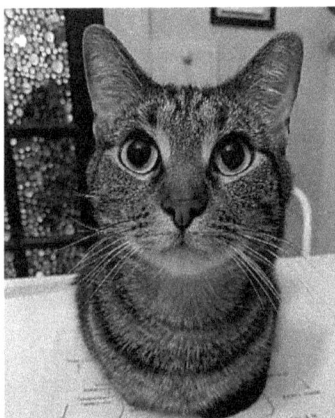

No, mental health is proactive. I am not tied to thinking in the same old way. Neither are you. Reframing thoughts and past experiences can serve to bring freedom to your present and future.

---

48 This is Ronan. He has suffered with fleas. It's no fun. You can follow him on Instagram at Ronan.thecat.sleeps

Chapter 19: Reframing the Past

Let's do a thought experiment. Look at your younger self. Look through your pictures, pick a few to talk to.

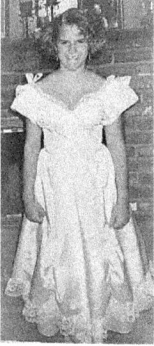

This is a picture of me the day I graduated 8th grade. This is the end of feeling fine about my body. The summer after this picture was taken, I started to put on weight.

The point of this thought experiment is to see what you think might have worked to put you on a different path with your relationship with food.

I realize this thought experiment is fraught. Some of you have come to your eating issues due to abuse or food insecurity as a child. Even though these experiences happen to us and shape us, we are ultimately free beings capable of change and hope. Peace to you.

Imagine for a moment your younger self made an appointment with you, looking for advice. What would you tell her? What would you tell the young you? What could you offer as a solution or range of solutions? How could you intervene in your younger life to have a different outcome with food?

I think the best approach would be to start with getting her talking. What is she thinking and feeling? What does she want to do with her life? What are her goals and dreams? What are her fears? What does she think it will take to live a good life?

I would ask questions for clarification. If her body image hadn't come up yet (and it wouldn't because I've always been a hider), I would ask her. I would ask her to trust me and tell me the truth. One thing I know about my teenage self is that I desperately wanted to be known, but I had to trust that the knower *really* wanted to know. I was a hard nut to crack.

Once I had this information, helping me to get back into the head of my younger self, I would identify the lies she is telling herself. The lie that she isn't good enough. The lie that the size of her body determines what she can do and whether she can be loved.

I would talk to my younger self about the constant and persistent lies of the beauty and consumerism industries. Since my younger self was bombarded with billion-dollar advertising campaigns designed to make her feel like crap, I would mount a full-fledged war against those poisonous ideas. I would have her watch documentaries like *MissRepresentation*. I would ask her why she thinks her destructive self-thoughts are true, and reinforce the truth that love is not dependent on body size.

How would I do this? Parade the number of thin-sized women who have been cheated on or passed over. Parade the number of plus-sized women who are in loving relationships (focusing here) and in positions of power.

I would tell her the truth about diets. Temporary restriction doesn't work. That's what a diet is. What is needed is a complete overhaul of how she views food, comfort, acceptance, and control. I would point to the recent studies that show adolescents on diets are astronomically more likely to develop eating disorders. I would tell her, myself – no diets.

The alternative I would offer her is finding healthy, lifelong coping mechanisms and learning about nutrition. I would recommend a year's worth of weekly visits with a nutritionist, counselor, and spiritual advisor. Each.

I would tell her no food is off limits. I would educate her on what food is for and how it can be her ally.

I would help her find healthy ways to find comfort, which is not in food.

I would ask her to journal about her feelings. I would then read the journals with her (with her permission) and talk to her about those feelings. Challenge the false ideas. Help her to see what was real and what wasn't.

I would help her to see her body as wonderful and a blessing. Something to cherish.

I would help her to see her worth is not dependent on what others think. Most of these "others" just want her money. Most of the "others," the marketing voices, see her as nothing more than an object to manipulate. They certainly don't have her best interests in mind.

I would break down magazine images for her. Teach her to recognize photoshop, hours in a make-up chair with professional make-up artists and beauticians. Help her to understand the lies a good photographer can pull off through the magic of lighting.

In an image focused world, I would challenge her to think about what's not in the frame posted. To have her verbally recognize how many shots it takes to get those perfect pictures. To humanize the celebrities. They are people and therefore have problems too.

End thought experiment

What I want for my younger self is to see herself clearly. What a wish!

Why is it we act against our own good? Why is it we can see how false images and a beauty-obsessed money-grubbing culture hates us, and how that culture destroys our friends and neighbors, but can't turn the insight around and apply it to ourselves?

It turns out I wanted my younger self to grow up in a culture that embraced and promoted healthy, life giving, and virtuous ideas. It looks like I wish my younger self lived in a utopia.

It is easy to give advice when you have unlimited imaginary resources to offer. My younger self needed intensive and sustained attention and therapy to train her on how and why to eat, how to understand her body, and how to see her worth.

The point of this thought experiment is mainly two-fold: to investigate my past to see how I can reframe some of my dysfunctional beliefs and to consider what could be changed in the present, so others may be less likely to fall into those traps.

There is no logical reason to keep us from changing our hostile culture. Our capitalist society is unwilling, currently. But it doesn't have to be this way. We can change our culture if we want. Given the body-positive push in the past few years, I have reason to hope we can turn the toxic culture around.

If we don't want to change the toxic culture that encourages eating disorders, obesity, and an overall general anxiety about our bodies not being good enough, I ask you, why? Why does this kind of fundamental change seem impossible? Why is it so radical to think of treating everyone, even children, with dignity and respect?[49]

---

[49] If we don't want to change the toxic culture that encourages eating disorders, obesity, and an overall general anxiety about our bodies not being good enough, I ask you, why? Why does this kind of fundamental change seem impossible? Why is it so radical to think of treating everyone, even children, with dignity and respect? Greed? Selfishness? Are these inborn or learned reactions to the world? Even if we are born with this kind of nature, can we model, expect, and train people to be kind to themselves and their neighbor? If not, why not? Why do we accept making a society toxic for the inhabitants and then blame them for not thriving?

Chapter 20: Food Addiction

Looking at the thought experiment in the previous chapter, I find it interesting what I left out. Food insecurity.

There was always food on my table. Fresh, homecooked food. I never went hungry as a child. On special occasions we went out to eat. Access to healthy foods was never an issue. The house was always stocked. Also, my parents loved me.

Why, then, do I fear lack of access to food? I think it's a control issue, which is, for many, at the root of food addiction. Ironic. When we are addicted, we are no longer in control. We've ceded control to the addiction. The addiction is in control, and we are along for the ride.

My lack of access to food hasn't been physical, but mental. Most of the foods I wanted to eat were no-no foods. Off limit foods. "Bad" foods.

I've never responded well to being told what to do. Admittedly, I have a problem with authority. Or at least, what I perceive as misplaced authority. I also have serious trust issues.

Someone wiser than me could probably put the pieces together regarding the origins of my food addiction. For some people, this kind of mental exercise of precisely putting the pieces of the past together to understand the present is essential in food addiction recovery. At present, I am fine with a fuzzy picture.

The theme that persists from my earliest malformed food relationship is about control. Who controls what I eat? Who controls who sees what I eat?

I figured out at an early age that could be me. I could control the extra food I ate by eating in secret.

When I ate and what I ate has been largely a struggle of control. I control what I eat, even if it disappoints the imagined "you." "You" make me feel bad for eating the junk food, so I

pretend in public to not be interested in what I really want –
one candy bar – and I buy more to prove I can do what I want.

It's the constant high of getting away with what I want. The
animal in the corner with her prize. My animal prize is usually
inordinate amounts of sugary treats.

At the end of college, I took a trip to Russia. I remember
being in the backseat of a taxi in Moscow, fearing for my life.
There were no traffic lines on the road and little discernable
rhythm or reason for the cars other than getting to your
destination as fast as you can. I was along for the ride, afraid
and fascinated. I didn't have enough confidence to stand up for
myself and what I thought was clearly dangerous and possibly
death inducing. While I wasn't actually a hostage, I felt
trapped.

This is how I think about food addiction: being in the back
of a taxi in a foreign city where you don't speak the language.

- *I got in the taxi because I thought it was a good idea.* I started
  eating to comfort myself. It tastes good. I like it. I'm in
  control.
- *Once in the taxi, I'm in the back and not steering.* At one
  point, I went from deciding to steal the cookies, to being
  compelled. I don't know when I moved from being in the
  driver's seat to the feeling of passenger. But it happened.
  Once the compulsion hit to eat high fat, high sugar,
  calorie packed foods, I was in the back for the ride.
- *The landscape is familiar in the sense of I know what cars are,
  what roads are, what buildings are, street signs. But I don't
  know these cars, roads, buildings, and I can't read the signs.* I
  was eating (familiar) but I knew I wasn't eating what I
  should've. My only food rule was to get what I want and
  satisfy the craving, regardless if it made me sick or was
  unhealthy.

- *I hear the taxi driver talking, asking questions, but I don't know what he's saying.* My passions were speaking, not my reason. It's like a haze continually clouding my mind, choking out the wise words of reason, turning her council to gibberish. The only voice I could hear was the devil's.
- *The taxi is zipping around in a way that feels death defying. I want out, but I don't know how to ask or how that would even work. If I got out in the middle of Moscow, what would I do next? Better stay in and chance it.* And this one is the kicker – the trap. What else was I supposed to do? What else was there? How else was I supposed to eat? How else could I live?

Somewhere in my early life I became a food addict. It may seem silly to talk about a food addiction because we all need food to live. In that sense, you might say we are "addicted" to food. But this, of course, is not what I mean when I say I'm a food addict.

What is addiction? Here are two definitions:

> Addiction is a treatable, chronic medical disease involving complex interactions among brain circuits, genetics, the environment, and an individual's life experiences. People with addiction use substances or engage in behaviors that become compulsive and often continue despite harmful consequences.[50]

> A compulsive, chronic, physiological, or psychological need for a habit-forming substance, behavior, or activity having harmful physical, psychological, or

---

[50] https://www.asam.org/Quality-Science/definition-of-addiction

social effects and typically causing well-defined symptoms (such as anxiety, irritability, tremors, or nausea) upon withdrawal or abstinence: the state of being addicted.[51]

One way to understand addiction is the loss of control. There are addictions that take us wholesale, and others in which we continue to be complicit. I've come to understand my food addiction as both.

There are times in my life when I feel completely lost and out of control.

It's like living with a manipulator. My addiction wants to manipulate and control me. I tried for years and years to deny it. To get past the addiction by calling it by a different name (laziness) and giving it a different diagnosis (lack of will power).

If you know anything about depression, you know you don't "will it" away. The problem is not the lazybones in the bed. The depressed person has a real malady that needs to be treated.

Depression is not addiction, so the parallel is not straight.

Food addiction dwells in an intersection where the amount of control a person has over the addiction shifts and changes.

In my experience, the addiction to eating and controlling what I ate had to do with "how good I was." I thought I was in charge and could get rid of the eating demon through rigorous self-control.

But this is not how treating eating addiction works – or, at least, not for me.

As with all addiction, recovery begins with admitting you have a problem, and you are powerless to solve it on your own. (See Appendix E)

---

[51] https://www.merriam-webster.com/dictionary/addiction

It wasn't until I acquiesced and admitted I was an addict that I could begin my journey towards making lasting peace with food.

The paradox again. To be free is to admit and embrace the lack of freedom.

I am an addict.

I will always be an addict.

Fine.

Next.

Once freed from the delusion I could shake the demon food addiction, I had a choice to make. Either allow it to run wild and let it continue to wreak havoc in my life or find another way.

The third way.

I do not give a damn that the science is out on food addiction. I mean, I love science. But, I don't need a person in a white coat telling me what is true about me. I also know that words are used in a variety of ways.[52]

Naming my condition as an addiction makes sense of my experience. It has helped me understand my struggle and given me a path forward.

Armed with this knowledge, moving forward, as far as I can see, involves the virtues. Developing the virtues, as Aristotle

---

[52] Addictions vary tremendously and cause different kinds of trauma to the people with the addiction and those who love and interact with them depending on the type of addiction (drugs, alcohol, sex, shopping, food, fame, etc.), the reasons for the addiction, and the way the person and society lives with and reacts to the addiction. By naming food addiction, I am calling out a real addiction even though it looks different from, say, the immediate destructiveness of a methamphetamine addiction. I see calling what I have an addiction as not only being wholly appropriate but stating a fact.

said, is the way towards human flourishing. I want to lead a flourishing human life.

Section III: Eating Addiction and the Virtues

Chapter 21: Food Addiction is Not a Moral Deficiency

Most of my life I saw being fat as a moral failing. I used to believe if I could just be good, I wouldn't be fat.

My sad, old thinking said to me:

- Fat is bad. Fat is within your control. You could easily be good by changing your eating habits. That you do not change your eating habits shows you are morally deficient.
- You lack the virtue of wisdom to know what to eat.
- You lack the virtue of justice to treat yourself with the proper dignity and respect.
- You lack moderation to eat the right amount at the right times.
- You lack courage to say 'no' to your desires to overindulge.

With this mentality I lived perpetually 'trying to be good' and failing. The failing was always in me. Always my fault. There was no one or thing to blame other than my own moral weakness.

I never stopped to question this theory. This was what I believed was true. But is it really accurate? Am I fat because I'm a bad person? Are there no other internal or external causes that are contributing to my inability to eat properly and maintain a healthy weight?

Once I began questioning my basic assumptions, **I found them to be false.**

A main factor in recovering from BED and living with my food addiction was a rejection of the lifelong dream I had to be thin. Once that was gone, I stopped looking at what I ate as either morally praiseworthy or morally degenerate. Honestly, once I stopped thinking about food, my internal morality food monitor went away.

Since I've started thinking about food again, I don't see eating as merely a moral issue. That's too simplistic (see chapter 16 for other causes). Why someone does or doesn't retain excess weight may or may not have to do with virtue or vice. May or may not. There is no way you can know from looking at a person if their weight, whatever it is, has to do with their moral condition.

I no longer believe my obesity is due to a simple moral deficiency on my part. I also firmly believe Aristotle is right: If you want to live a happy and healthy life, you need to be virtuous. Virtue, according to Aristotle in his *Nicomachean Ethics*, is acting according to the golden mean in the situation you are in:

Virtue, then, is a state of character concerned with choice, lying in a mean, i.e., the mean relative to us, this being determined by a rational principle by which the [person] of practical wisdom would determine it. Now it is a mean between two vices, that which depends on excess and that which depends on defect; and again it is a mean because the vices respectively fall short of or exceed what is right in both passions and actions, while virtue finds and chooses that which is intermediate.

So, what does virtue look like when you have a food addiction? Can I still seek virtue even though I'm an addict? The answer is an unequivocal yes! While there are loads of virtues, let's look at the four cardinal (first) virtues of wisdom, moderation, courage, and justice in relation to food addiction.

Chapter 22: Wisdom

What wisdom is

The person who is wise has insight into the world. She can look at a situation and sum it up accurately. She has a penetrating gaze into the way things are. The wise person has knowledge, experience, and moral goodness. The wise are who we go to for advice and are the ones we trust.

What wisdom is not

Wisdom is not the same as knowledge. Just because you know something, or a lot of things, doesn't make you wise. Do you know anyone with a Ph.D. who lacks common sense? Do you know anyone who never went to college and is yet the wisest person you've ever met? It is not enough to know about the world, you need to be able to apply your knowledge in everyday living.

But wisdom isn't just about applying knowledge. The bank robbing safe cracker can apply her knowledge to breaking into safes, but is she wise? No, for she lacks moral goodness. Moral goodness is key to being wise.

The wise person is not arrogant or needing of the spotlight. She does not lord her wisdom over others but shares her insights when appropriate, lovingly, and without pomp and circumstance.

Wisdom is the mother virtue needed in order to have any of the other virtues. How can you be courageous, self-controlled, moderate, patient, or loving if you are not first of all wise?

Know thyself

Wisdom involves knowing yourself. What does it mean to really know yourself? You say, "Merry, I've lived with myself my entire life, of course I know myself!"

Walker Percy wrote a fabulous book entitled *Lost in the Cosmos*. In it he includes these questions and observations about the self:

> You have seen yourself a thousand times in the mirror, face to face. No sight is more familiar. Yet why is it that the first time you see yourself in a clothier's triple mirror – from the side, so to speak – It comes as a shock? Or the first time you saw yourself in a home movie; were you embarrassed? What about the first time you heard your recorded voice – did you recognize it? Clearly, you should since you've been hearing it all your life.
>
> Why is it that, when you are shown a group photograph in which you are present, you always (and probably covertly) seek yourself out? To see what you look like? Don't you know what you look like? …
>
> One of the peculiar ironies of being a human self in the Cosmos: A stranger approaching you in the street will in a second's glance see you whole, size you up, place you in a way in which you cannot and never will, even though you spent a lifetime with yourself, live in the Century of the Self, and therefore ought to know yourself best of all.

It's not as easy to really know yourself as you might think. Consider your relationship with food. Explain to me why you eat what you eat. Don't skip this exercise. I encourage you to pause to spend time and sum up the whys of what you eat. Go ahead. Put down this book and write out your answer.

Even though I think I overeat because I primarily love the taste and feeling of food, I know I also eat because I'm bored, tired, stressed, sad, feel loss of control, and out of habit. But still I ask, why? My reason tells me if I eat whatever I want I won't be healthy. Eating in wild abandon is counter to my desires to be healthy and live at a reasonable weight.

Then why? Why do I still want to hold on to this aberrant and destructive behavior? I'm reminded of what St. Paul asks about his own actions in his letter to the Romans – Why do I do the evil I don't want to do and not the good I want to do?[53]

I used to think wisdom in relation to my food addiction was admitting, embracing, and conquering my lack of self-control.

I was wrong.

To truly know myself when it comes to disordered eating, the "easy" route is just to say the problem is me. I'm just weak and not wise enough.

While this way of thinking is appealing because it's clear-cut and fits with what society thinks, it isn't wise. The reasons I am addicted to food are many. It isn't simply the issue of lack of wisdom. Truly knowing myself is knowing, understanding, and facing why I do what I do. Taking the appropriate responsibility, but not more than I should. No less and no more.

Wisdom requires understanding the causes and reasons of my disorder and acting accordingly. Here is my **very unscientific** pie chart of the causes and reasons of my eating addiction:

---

[53] Romans 7:15

My eating addiction causes

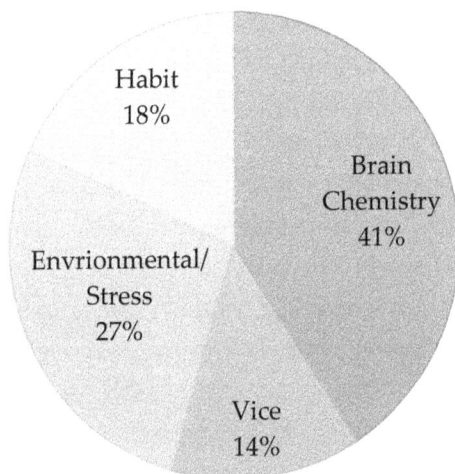

Habit
18%

Brain
Chemistry
41%

Envrionmental/
Stress
27%

Vice
14%

Wowzah! Would you look at that! When I look at this pie chart, I see my lack of virtue is only a small portion of why I eat the way I do. Does this let me off the moral hook? No. It lets me properly see its role, so I can act. Wisdom shows me what to do and what to address. When I wrongly assumed eating was simply a moral failing that was the only antidote. Be better.

I now see I have various issues I need to address. The more I grow in wisdom, I can imagine my pie chart becoming clearer. The sharper the problems are, the clearer the solutions. How can you solve a problem when you don't really know what the problem is? Wisdom is empowering and leads to action.

Chapter 23: Moderation

What moderation is

Moderation is a virtue concerned with the passions. The moderate person is able to fill the appetites of the body properly, giving the body what it needs. It finds the middle ground between what is too much and what is not enough.

The moderate person sees physical pleasure as a good to be protected and used when appropriate. The moderate person does not always hold physical pleasure at bay but engages in the bodily pleasures in the right way. Because the moderate person knows how to enjoy pleasure, she does not overindulge. She knows when to say 'no' to the pleasures of food, sex, and drink, and when to say 'yes' and in the proper quantity.

When it comes to eating, moderation has to do with properly dealing with the body's desires for food. What moderation looks like for each individual is going to vary significantly.

It is not moderate to live on less than 800 calories a day (if you have more food available to you). It is also not moderate to consume more than 3,000 calories a day (unless you are an Olympic swimmer or have some unusual dietary need). The moderate person knows how much she needs to eat and stays within that range. This is not to say the moderate person never enjoys a feast – she does … just not every day, and at every meal.

The moderate person is in control of her food choices and chooses those pleasures that are consistent with the flourishing life.

What moderation is not

Moderation is not mediocrity, being uptight, or giving the body all it wants. It is not about simply denying the body of physical pleasure for the sake of denial. The immoderate person sees pleasure as the ultimate good at one extreme or to be completely avoided at the other end of the scale.

Sometimes we praise the person who completely abstains from bodily pleasure, admiring her for her disdain of the body. Sometimes we praise the person we consider liberated, who is uninhibited and follows her lusts. But these models of defect and excess are not healthy.

Our bodies are good. Moderation helps us see pleasure for what it is, and for what it is not. We should partake in the pleasures of the body, but not as the purpose of all our actions. Physical pleasure is good, but it is not the only good. When we see and seek physical pleasure moderately, we become free to experience physical pleasure intentionally, completely, and not as tainted by inordinate passions that want us to over (or under) indulge.

Striving for moderation

When I first started thinking about what moderation with food looked like, I decided it was not possible for me to be moderate with food. There were some foods that were too powerful for me to consume in moderation. On my Last Diet Ever I decided, since I was addicted to sugar, I couldn't have it. I concluded, just as the alcoholic can't drink in moderation, the person addicted to sugar can't have it in moderation.

Unfortunately, it was this way of thinking that contributed to my binge eating disorder and depression. I was wound so tight, it's no wonder I snapped. I restricted, restricted, restricted until the dam broke, leaving my mental resources depleted and me completely shattered. If you want to see a dismal picture of a person desperately trying to be virtuous through restriction, I refer you to Appendix C, which is a 30-day peek into a woman who was in the grips of trying incredibly hard to conquer her sugar demon – no, who thought she had conquered him. One only needs to read to see she is very ill.

The following is what I wrote about moderation when I was on my Last Diet Ever. When I wrote this, I was still months away from snapping.

I have faced facts. I am a food-aholic. I love food too much. I am broken when it comes to food, and I wish, to this day, I never had to eat again. The alcoholic loves alcohol, is drawn to alcohol, and is destroyed by her love. I love food and it both nourishes and poisons me. The alcoholic must leave her love behind and never have it again, EVER. This is very harsh, but the only way. There is not a moderate way for alcoholics to drink alcohol. They are broken and cannot have another drink if they want to be free from living drunk or living to drink.

When I picture a moderate person's relationship with sweets, I imagine the person who has a dessert once or twice a week. Maybe the moderate person has a bag of mini chocolate bars she keeps in her desk at work, or in the kitchen, and eats one or two a day. The moderate person goes to a party and might sample a few of the desserts there. On occasion she might order something decadent from her favorite restaurant.

My goal is to be a moderate eater. I would love to be rightly related to sweets, so I could enjoy the occasional piece of birthday cake or outing to Baskin Robins. However, this is not possible for me.

I had to realize, for me, sugar is a drug. It calls my name. Once I start, I find it nearly impossible to stop. What do I get out of one piece of birthday cake? First, I want to make certain I get a large piece, with extra frosting. As I'm eating my first piece, I'm sizing up the situation to see how likely it is that I can have a second, maybe a third.

I decided if I really wanted to live as a free person I had to stop, totally, the consumption of all things candy. No more Jr. Mints, ice cream, brownies, baklava, cookies, cakes, frosting, Rice Krispies Treats, mochas, and the list streams on infinitely.

Why would I decide to be so immoderate? Because I have tried to peacefully co-exist with having treats in my life, but they always end up getting the better of me. I cannot make it work. I am not like my mother-in-law who can bake delicious cookies (without eating the cookie dough) and eat ONE cookie! No good comes out of me eating a cookie. No good. One cookie is never enough, and neither are ten.

***

What do I understand the virtue of moderation to be now? I understand moderation to be eating the right amount at the right time for the right reasons, *as one is able*.[54]

What is different for me now goes to the paradox: I thought my addiction to sugar would be solved by leaving it behind completely. The opposite was true, for me. When I gave up ENTIRELY on restricting, the appeal and worry of eating sugar subsided. Sugar lost its death grip because I stopped playing the-tug-of-war with it.

I am doing surprisingly well. When I embraced my no-diets ever mindset, the allure of sugar fell away, for years and years.

When I started taking weight loss medicine, my old killer thoughts resurfaced, but once the medicine settled in I found it calms my mind, so that eating/not eating isn't constantly running on a loop in my mind. I also found I rarely overeat. In addition to not constantly thinking about food, I get full and sick to my stomach if I eat too much.

Even though I'm on weight loss medicine, sometimes I just want to eat and eat (stress and emotional eating), and I eat (because of my mantra). Nine times out of 10, I pay the price of

---

[54] *As one is able* is my new caveat. Moderation is not all or nothing. There is the ideal of moderate eating, but for the broken, the ideal is unlikely to be met. The good news is the virtue of moderation is relative to the person. Moderation for me, given my food addiction, is different from those with no eating issues.

feeling sick to my stomach for the rest of the evening. The best way for me to describe it is akin to natural and logical consequences. I have been burned enough times to think twice about putting my hand to the fire. The reaction, the nausea, quickly follows overeating. When I look at the food now, I ask myself, "Is *it* worth it?" The *it* is the sickness. For someone who has control issues with food, the short clear path from overeating to feeling sick helps me to say 'no.' The long path of "overeating may cause all of these health issues leading to possible early death" is what I know intellectually. But the long path doesn't seem to matter when the food is right in front of me. What does matter is whether I'm going to be sick for the rest of the evening. I seem to be able to decide to stop eating because I don't want the consequence of that immediate effect.

I've had practice with immediate consequences and alcohol. For a while now, when I drink more than likely I will wake up with a headache, and I mean one glass of wine will do this to me.

I've tried loads of remedies to prevent the morning-after headache such as: drinking lots of water all day and after the wine consumption; not drinking on an empty stomach; and drinking imported wine to avoid the chemical in the American bottling system.

All without success. Thus, I've learned. I ask myself, "Do you really want to wake with a headache? Is this glass of wine really worth feeling like crap the next day?" I'm now down to drinking a glass every four months or so … just to test it. So far, the same result: Headache.

I've found moderation in the most unlikely of places: non-restriction and modern science.

I first found moderation through giving up on restriction. I ate what I wanted, when I wanted, and went on with my daily business freed from the constant tyranny of my food addiction.

When my aging body changed and I began to gain weight I felt uncomfortable with, I found moderation through medicine. This, for me, feels like a miracle. The medicine has cleared the haze of my food frenzy. I still have to repeat my mantra, "I'm not on a diet. I can eat what I want," when the food crazy calls to me. But now, thanks to the calming of my brain, I feel I can make decisions about what is and isn't too much to eat.[55]

As I've mentioned before, I entirely plan to stay medicated the rest of my life, if possible. While I have work to do in the area of moderation with my food, I am further along than I thought possible. I eat whatever I want and when I want. I eat all the sugar I want. I eat all the fast-food I desire. While I heartily acknowledge fast-foods and their kin are not healthy to eat (in general), this is where I see the possibility for personal

---

[55] While in the process of editing this book, I went on a small vacation to visit extended family. Being out of my normal routine and not in control of the "whats" and "whens" of eating still makes me anxious. I found myself eating to the point of sickness. The medicine lets me know when I overeat and kicks me in the stomach. The threat of feeling bad is usually enough, lately, for me not to overindulge. But not on this vacation. I "pushed-through" the sickness because I wanted to eat. I needed to eat. I was stressed out trying to manage everyone's emotions. Guess what? My family is lovely. Guess what? No one needs me to manage their emotions. The problem is entirely with me. But I still feel that burden of trying to make everything smooth and conflict free.

All of this to say, to date, the medicine usually helps me to eat moderately. When, however, I find myself under specific situations where I feel out of control, I tend to eat too much. The medicine hasn't brought complete moderation. I see room for improvement in this area using different techniques, such as being honest with my family about my food anxiety and addiction, consulting a therapist, etc.

growth in becoming moderate. And yet, this is tricky for me since I will **not** restrict my food intake. I am a work in progress.

Chapter 24: Justice

What justice is

Justice is fairness and giving people their due. The just are concerned with treating others the way they deserve to be treated. All people deserve to be regarded in a fair manner and this is what the just person does. She does not play favorites when it comes to doling out justice, but is impartial and evenhanded.

One representation of justice in the U.S. legal system is of a woman blindfolded holding scales. She symbolizes rewards and punishments based on merit, not vindictiveness, favoritism, or the desire to make someone an "example" to the community.

An important Greek philosopher, Plato, concludes in his great work the *Republic* that justice in the ideal society is everyone doing their job (what they ought) and minding their own business. The just tend to their own needs and place in society (not slacking-off but being a contributing member of the community) and leave others to do the same. We might say today the just aren't micromanagers, but rather they let each person do what he or she is supposed to.

Ideal societies and actual societies are quite a bit different, yet it is important to see what justice should be in order to try and realize this great goal; for we all want peace in the world, as we want it in our own homes, as we want it with food. If we neglect justice, we get war.

What justice is not

The excess of justice is revenge. When someone hurts us, we desire to strike back. Retaliation usually ends in escalation: you push me, I hit you, you stab me, I shoot you. Revenge has us seeking not an eye for an eye but a head for an eye.

Justice distributes punishment according to the severity of the crime committed, as informed by the intellect, whereas vengeance is always fueled by passion with little to no reflection or reason.

The defect of justice is an apathetic concern for the rights of others. The person with this defect does not diligently seek the restoration of what is lost or taken from another. She might tell all a particular set of rules and in the end disregard them, turning all who participated into "winners."

Think of the person who works her tail off to win the science fair prize or get the promotion at work. You know that many others worked half-heartily to win the prize or achieve the promotion. When the time comes for the winner to be announced how would that person feel if the science panel said, "We've decided all who entered a project are winners regardless of the actual worth of their project." How would a person feel if her boss decided all were to be "promoted" even though most did nothing to merit the promotion? It is deflating to work towards a goal only to be told your hard work is of no consequence. The person who lacks justice does not see (or care) that disregarding the rules is unfair, demoralizing, and counterproductive.

Shame

When I think of the children starving in the world, I am ashamed. I am ashamed that one of my major failings is I have too much food and can't seem to control myself. I am blessed to live in a country overflowing with milk and honey. I am immensely grateful I don't have to worry about where my next meal is coming from or whether I'll be able to feed my children, though, of course, even in the United States families go to bed hungry more than I'd like to admit or think about.

When I was volunteering in my child's classroom for a class party, several of the kindergarten teachers decided to order McDonald's food for the kids. By the time the food was delivered it was less than tasty - have you ever eaten cold McDonald's French fries? As I was cleaning up, I noticed my son's teacher putting some left-over hamburgers and fries in a child's backpack. She saw me watching her and explained if she didn't send this food home the child might not eat tonight. This tiny kindergartner in my town – hungry.

Is there justice in the world?

If justice is giving each what is owed, then there is no perfect justice in the world. How can you repay the fire fighter who risks her life to save your child? How can a murderer pay for what she has done? Perfect justice is not to be had in this life.

If the ideal of justice cannot be, should justice still be sought after? Of course. If we want peace, we must fight for justice. The slogan "No justice, no peace" is true. When people are taken advantage of civil unrest and war are the natural reactions. We will only attain peace, the state we all desire when we fight for justice and bring it about as much as possible.

When I think of the injustice in the world, I am overwhelmed. I am tempted to fall into despair and conclude that nothing can be done to bring about justice so why try.

Justice begins with each person doing what they ought. You do the right thing regardless of the decisions of others.

Is it just that I have had these tortuous eating issues? Is it just that I have never gone hungry a day in my life because my family isn't poor? No. This is luck or providence. I don't deserve to live in the time and country that is mine. It is not owed to me to hail from a family that has access to food and clean water.

Justice and food addiction

Years ago, when I thought about the relationship between food addiction and justice, I mistakenly thought I would conquer my inordinate eating through food restriction. This is what I wrote:

That I might have a genetic predisposition to hoard food, love sugar, not feel satiated is beside the point.

Justice in my food life is not about what was given to me through nature *but what I do with the nature I have.*

I am disordered and it is up to me to find a way to come out of the chaos. I must find a way to be just and treat my body fairly. Justice in eating for me means (1) Eating enough food every day – not too much and not too little; (2) filling my body with good, high-quality foods such as fruits, veggies, dairy, good fats; (3) finding a way to avoid unnecessary abstinence; (4) and embracing this body I have.

For a while I was eating too much Kashi cereal. It turns out my excessive eating of this cereal did not usually result in me going over my allotted calories for the day. However, this cereal made me feel out of control because I ate more of it than I had originally given myself permission.

I thought about why I couldn't seem to get enough of this cereal and concluded I liked it because it's sweet. My first reaction was to add this cereal to my banned food list.

It is hard for me to enjoy my food now. I feel if I'm enjoying what I'm eating I must be doing something wrong. I'm afraid if I like it, I'm leading myself down the garden path to eating inordinately, hiding in a closet somewhere with a fist full of cookies.

The fact of the matter is I am a physical creature with a body and, gasp, taste buds. I need to learn it is okay to enjoy the food I am eating, and it is okay to feel full. Learning to accept the fleshiness of human existence is a challenge when I've fought my body for so many years. You are human too, flesh and bone. (I decided not to exile Kashi to my banned food list.)

***

Though I wrote of acceptance, I didn't really mean it. I thought justice was the judge, fairly labeling my desire to eat as unhinged and therefore to be rooted out. But I was wrong. Justice, in relation to food addiction, is treating the body and mind fairly. It is just to assess what is really going on instead of looking at the symptoms (food consumption) of the disorder. It is just to treat the addiction, and unjust to ignore it. If you treat the addiction, you are on your way to making peace with food, both internally and externally. If you ignore your food addiction and continue to mislabel it as "undisciplined eating," you will stay in a perpetual state of warring against yourself.

Justice without mercy is deadly

Even when I was wrong about what justice was in relationship to living with a food addiction, I was crying out for mercy and understanding. Unfortunately, at the time, I was anything but merciful to myself. I was cruel and acted the villain. A part of recovering from binge eating disorder was when I began to see myself as deserving of mercy. I deserve mercy and so do you.

I was showing myself no mercy because I was disregarding the external and internal factors that led to my food addiction. Look at my unjust sugar restriction. I basically told myself, you break the rules and you die. There are no extenuating circumstances to hear and no second chances.

How would you like your justice system to operate? Should all be treated alike with the sword, or should we listen to the circumstances of the individual and dole out justice *and* mercy?

When you assess your eating disorder, treat yourself justly. See what you deserve. You are a human and therefore first of all deserve to be treated with dignity and respect. As you judge your past and present eating mistakes, see clearly and wisely the damage you have done (not overstating the case), but don't serve yourself justice without it being tempered with the salve of mercy.

Chapter 25: Courage

What courage is
Courage curbs inordinate fears. When threatened with pain, physically or psychologically, courage is needed to face the situation and act according to reason, not misguided passion. When you are courageous you stand firm in your rational beliefs, even in the face of fear. Fear tries to pull us away from how we know we ought to act. Wisdom tells us what to do in a situation and courage enables us to carry out the dictates of reason.

Years ago, I reasoned courage in relation to food addiction was the ability to stand firm in my convictions that I couldn't eat sugar, and that I had to tightly watch everything that entered my mouth. I was mistaken. Here's an excerpt from what I *thought* courage meant:

When you know what you should eat, the virtue of courage fortifies you, giving you the ability to say no to your cravings.

When I am at a movie theater my reason tells me to stay away from the large tub of buttered popcorn, soda, and Reese's Pieces. My reason tells me, but do I have the courage to stand up to my appetites?

Have you ever been bullied? Remember what it feels like to have someone intimidate you, to feel fear for your safety or livelihood? The virtue of courage is needed to stand up to the bully – to turn her in to the authorities or reject her commands.

When you are ruled by your appetites, they become like the bully on the playground, pushing you around, taking your lunch money, giving you a black eye. A bully stares you down and expects you to give into her demands.

The virtue of courage lets you look the appetite bully in the metaphorical eye and refuse to give in. The appetite bully spares no expense and pulls all the punches. She says, "But you'll miss out if you don't. You'll be sad if you don't. You'll be hungry if you don't. People will laugh at you if you don't. People will be disappointed in you if you don't. This is the only chance you'll get to eat."

Courage helps you stand your ground as your appetites try to seduce you away.

***

This view of courage is **shallow**. I used to think my food addiction was simple: You eat too much. Stop eating too much. Therefore, with this wrong-headed understanding of the problem, I'm not surprised I misunderstood the work of the virtues in relation to my problem.

Courage is still the mean between excess and deficiency, but the golden mean I seek is now internal and not what I put in my mouth. I now see the role of courage is to deal with the addiction itself, not the symptoms.

What courage is not

Courage isn't being fool hearty. The person with the excess of courage is reckless. She calls it bravery, but it is nothing other than foolishness to run head-long into dangerous situations unnecessarily.

Courage isn't cowardice. The coward runs away from fearful situations. She runs and hides until it is safe to come out. The coward does and says whatever her fears tell her to do. She is not free to live as she desires.

Yet again, I misunderstood cowardice in relationship to food.

Imagine going into battle. Your squad is lined up and waiting for the commander's call to charge. The foolhardy person rushes to the battle (and almost certain death) before the commander has blown the horn. Once the horn is blown, the coward turns around and heads for the trees, toward safety. The person with courage stays and fights the battle.

Now imagine going to a 4th of July party. What's on the menu? A variety of BBQ meats, grandma's potato salad, chips galore, and all manner of desserts.

The coward gives into her fears, unable to say 'no' to the powerful tempter. The foolhardy person takes no precautions, such as eating before the party, making an eating plan and/or bringing healthy foods to eat. What happens to her? She easily succumbs to the power of her appetites.

The person with courage is steadfast. She knows what awaits her at the buffet line. She knows her appetites are there, lying in wait to ambush her efforts. She sees and stands her ground – staring her opponent down. She has the courage to say no to her appetites who so desperately want multiple helpings of chocolate cake, homemade ice cream, and Uncle Sammy's famous BBQ ribs. The courageous person emerges from the food war as the victor.

***

This is the picture of a psyche wound so tight, it's no wonder I flew apart. I thoroughly believed I was in a war, and I needed the warrior's courage to defeat the enemy of my nemesis, food. But that was misplaced courage. True courage is embracing reality and continuing to act for the good. I'd invested so much of myself into this idea of conquering my food demons, I wasn't open to the possibility that fighting with myself had nothing to do with courage or cowardice.

I've found courage in relation to my food addiction is not about attacking myself about what I eat, but about coming to terms with acknowledging my addiction. I lived in self-deceit, ignorant of my real condition. For me, someone with a food addiction, courage is acknowledging my disorder to myself and others, not hiding. Courage is the willingness not to try to reason with my addicted food mindset. Courage is not found in standing up to the internal food crazy thoughts, but rather walking forward and looking for ways to deal with my condition, even if those ways are scary. Courage is extracting myself from the position of demanding to have the ability to "win" against my appetites and deciding not to play along, but seek help instead.

Of all of the virtues, courage I lack most of all. I find it difficult to be honest with myself and the world. I have an overwhelming inner monologue, so many feelings and thoughts about the nature of existence, society, and the problem of evil.

I am convinced virtue is the right path for all of us. If you want a good human life, virtue is the way to human happiness. Notice that one important aspect of virtue ethics is the particularity of it. Virtue is always the mean between the two extremes of excess and defect, but where that mean is lies relative to the particular circumstances in which someone finds themselves. In every circumstance, the golden mean (human excellence) can be found.

How can we know what the golden mean is given the situation we find ourselves? Aristotle claims the person with practical wisdom will know the mean. The person who is wise is the one who can find the virtue sweet spot between the extremes. I'm therefore not surprised I misunderstood the relationship of food to virtue. While I know I'm not wise now, when I originally wrote on the virtues, I was self-deceived about my condition, its cause, and its cure.

And now? I feel I'm closer to understanding what a virtuous relationship looks like for me and my particular circumstances. I am and will always be a food addict. Therefore, for me, a virtuous relationship with food respects that fact, acknowledges it, and works with the addiction to make peace with food.

SECTION IV: MOVING FORWARD

Chapter 26: Making Peace with My Body

As I came out of the haze of BED, I developed my plan for a food restriction-free life. This meant the body I had would be it. Once I came to terms with the fact that I was going to be overweight forever, I chose to embrace the body I had, not the one I longed to have. This was part of the healing. The only reasons I had to not love my body was due to false internalized messages about what is beautiful and worthy.

I decided to dress the body I had.

I've always liked clothes. I love color, texture, and pattern. I'm such a sucker for design and creativity. Seeing beautiful textiles brings me joy.

It's not that one day I was wearing rags and the next I was glammed up. My entire adult life I've had the tendency to overdress. What changed was what I was trying to achieve.

Since my early teen years, I used clothes as a security blanket in which to hide from myself and others. Maybe I could feel better about myself if what I was wearing was pretty or cool, even if I weren't.

In 2003, *What Not to Wear* debuted on TLC. I remember scoffing at the premise. Take some poorly dressed, shlumpy woman (usually), shame her, throw ALL her clothes away in front of her and the world to see, give her $5,000 for a new wardrobe, and finish her off with a make-up and hair makeover.

I mean, have you ever heard of something more materialistic and awful? But … I watched. My husband and I tuned in regularly. What I found was something very different from what I imagined.

Transformation.

Stacy and Clinton (the hosts) were telling people to dress the body they currently had, not the one they wanted or had in the past. You deserve to feel good because you deserve to feel good in your body. They preached the message of embracing who you are today, right now. Feeling good and embracing your body doesn't need to wait until you've lost that "tummy" you've been hiding or until you shed those baby pounds.

Through this show I began to see other women feel good about themselves, even though they usually weren't the smaller size they wanted to be. It turned out, the week the contestants spent in New York with the hosts and staff of *What Not to Wear* worked as a kind of personal rehab. You could see it on their faces. Most went kicking and screaming into the show, only to embrace the process on the other end.

Through this show, I heard for the first time that when something doesn't fit, it's not your fault – it's the clothes. In other words, there is nothing wrong with my body. If the clothes don't fit, there's something wrong with them (and/or the manufacturers). The clothes are wrong for me because they don't fit me. I'm not wrong because I don't fit them.

This sounds basic, but I tucked that idea away. I also took seriously the size of my current body and began looking for clothes that were made for my shape. It doesn't matter what the fad of the time is, what matters is embracing and dressing the shape you have.

I embraced A-line dresses! My wardrobe is filled with them.

I was watching *What Not to Wear* during my normal vicious cycle of diet failures. I started looking to dress the body I had, still holding on to the "someday thin" clothes. Once I was on the road to recovery from BED, I got rid of them. All of them. I saw "thin" clothes as nothing but mental baggage.

I acknowledged I would not be that weight again.

Acceptance.

I acknowledged I had the body I had.

Acceptance.

My body, my obese body, was mine. And in this body, I did really great things! Once I really, truly, embraced my body at 190 pounds, I found peace and my focus shifted.

In general, I'm a grateful person. I feel I have an abundance of blessings. A husband who loves me, three great kids, a lovely house, a loving family. I've never lacked for any need.

Once I accepted my body as-is, I started to be thankful for all it gave me such as this wonderful life it allowed me to live. I found myself being thankful my body worked as it did.

At this time, I was a lecturer of philosophy at the University of Tennessee at Martin. As I looked at my sea of students, I wanted them to be successful and whole people. I began to shift my focus from what I had been wearing as a cover-up for an unacceptable body to that of a role-model. I could use my wardrobe to send a message to those of all weights that a woman who is obese can be a professional. Your size is irrelevant. I doubt anyone on the outside of my head noticed this shift, but I did.[56] This shift in thinking from hiding my body to dressing as a role model for others was immeasurably beneficial to the peace I made with food.

Making peace with food came in respecting and not denying my food addiction. It's there, I just deflated its power.

> **Problem 1**: The food addiction is at its most powerful when I restrict my food intake.
> **Solution:** Don't restrict. Don't get in a pissing contest with a water tower.

---

[56] I admit I worried I had this new shift of thought to justify spending money on a wardrobe. As with many endeavors, our motivations are plural. It can be distressing not to think and act out of a singular motivation; welcome to the human mind. Why we do and think as we do often has a variety of causes and motivations.

Problem 2: Believing my body is bad because it's fat.
Solution: Your body is your body. Seek to change your thinking and embrace, accept, and dress the body you have.

Paying attention to how I look, and seeing myself as a role model to other people, dispersed the obsession of 'thin is good.'

How do you treat your body? Think about the amount of mental energy you spend thinking about food. Now, compare that to the time and attention you pay to dressing your body. Why do you wear the clothes you wear?

On the point of how to dress your body, we vary as to how much we care about aesthetics and to what we find aesthetically pleasing. Some of you would never wear a dress regardless of your body size because you don't like dresses. Some of you would never put on a pair of leggings because you think they are hideous.

I am not making some grand statement that making peace with food is about dressing up and being a clothes horse like me. However, I do think it is foolish to neglect the effect of the external physical world on the mind.

Plato was right when he claimed what we experience externally in our environment gives us clues as to how to act and what to expect.

Imagine you are taking a class at a university. You walk into the lecture hall and it's clear the room hasn't been cleaned in a while. There is trash piled up high above and spilling over the rim of the trashcan. Half of the overhead lights are out. The few that are on are blinking. You take a seat, sweating already because it's the dead of summer and the air isn't on. You see a rat scurry by out of the corner of your eye as the professor enters. She's dressed in what is clearly a swimsuit cover up, curlers in her hair, and a cigarette dangling out of the side of her mouth.

Given this environment, do you really expect anything serious or of importance to take place? The environment says the university doesn't think whatever is going on here is important and neither should you.

Our environments give us clues as to what is happening and what is and isn't expected of us. This holds true for how we dress our bodies. Think about your pandemic experience. Many of us had the experience of showering less, dressing down, and/or not getting out of pjs. Think about how it feels to be dressed up, whatever that means to you. How do you feel and what kinds of things do you do? Consider what it feels like to be dressed up vs. in sleeping clothes. I by no means think everyone experiences the world as I do. But when I don't shower and wear my paint-stained raggedy leggings, I've told myself I'm not doing much. Not going out. Not working on anything, other than making it through my backlog of whatever I've currently recorded on my DVR.

It's the middle of June, I've recently quit my job, and I'm all dressed up and at a local coffee shop. I did my hair, make-up, etc. because if I don't get ready for the day in this way, the chances of me accomplishing anything of importance is extremely low.

When I tell myself the body I have is important and worthy of attention, my mind gets this idea too. For me, one way to get this message into my brain is through paying attention and taking care of what I wear. After my Last Diet Ever, I couldn't look at myself in a full-length mirror. I hated my body. Or rather, I hated the defeat the fat represented.

As I healed from the disappointment and BED, my mind cleared. I found myself able to take the sight of me without wincing. Slowly, I saw myself as a person with a particular body, not a hideous failure. Nothing really changed on the outside, but when I let go of ever dieting and resigned myself to the current size of my body, the most amazing thing happened: I began to like what I saw.

When I look in the mirror now, sometimes I am amazed at how pretty I think I am. I can't believe I've just admitted this, but it's true. When I look in the mirror, I see my pretty hazel eyes, my interesting complexion, and my curves. I look down and I like my hands. When I'm naked, I like my shape. It's not only cozy, but it's me. Sometimes I'll poke and prod the fat and wonder why I cared so much. Wonder why I think if it melted away, my life would be radically better.

The fact of the matter is that if someone wants to find fault with you, they will. It doesn't really matter what you look like. The famous and "beautiful" in our culture are routinely picked on, bullied, and dragged through the mud. I had a friend in college who was beautiful, Barbie beautiful. Guess what? She was hated and adored for her beauty. She was abused by a lover. I saw her beauty as a blessing and a curse.

But that's all of us. The size of your body, the sound of your voice, your height, your societal status, whatever you are that others see from the outside can be blessings and curses. The difference comes from how we think about ourselves.

For example, I'm 5'1" tall. I'm on the shorter side. Some might say short. How do I feel about my height? I don't feel a thing about it. Could I feel proud or embarrassed by my height? Sure. But I don't. I don't think about my height, that is until I stand side-by-side with my six-foot-tall husband. That is about the only time I feel short. But even that feeling of shortness doesn't feel bad, but more like a matter of fact.

My mind has transitioned to seeing my body in much the same way. A fact. I am the weight that I am. I have the rolls that I have. The only one who can really make me feel bad (or good!) about my weight is me. If someone else tries to make me feel bad about my weight, the very fact of their trying cannot make me feel bad. I mean, if someone tried to fat shame me to my face, the problem is clearly with the shamer and not with me.

But, as we know, a lot of fat shaming doesn't come in that personal way. Fat shaming is just in the air we breathe with the fat jokes, unavailable clothes and bra sizes, small chairs, lack of representation, diet culture, etc.

I get to decide how to think about my body. For me, I have this power (and it does feel like power … almost a superpower!) because I'm off the diet mentality. I am done with it. Its threat is no longer hanging over my head. I'm out and its power is gone.

Chapter 27: Love and Acceptance

I wasted much of my life living with the pain of the FALSE belief that fat is bad, ugly, and unlovable.

To be fat with these false beliefs in a thin-loving world is to live with chronic disappointment and despair. Fat is visual. Everywhere you go, there are eyes. Most of us go about our lives thinking people experience the world in much the way we do. If you ask anyone to examine that default, unconscious assumption, fairly quickly they'd see this belief as untrue.

But this evil, insidious belief of "fat is awful and so are you" was ever present for twenty-five years of my life, most pronounced in my teenage and young adult years.

For decades, I walked around with the baggage of thinking I was being constantly sized up by strangers' eyes and deemed expendable, uninteresting, and lazy. Walking down the aisle in a grocery store, walking through the mall, sitting in class, everywhere I went this belief haunted me.

A real haunting. This belief was just, I thought, because I deserved to be judged, shamed, and punished because I was bad. Clearly, I was bad because I was fat.

I am not a good enough writer to convey how it feels to be living in your own skin that you truly think is bad. How do I explain the constant barrage of negative thoughts that ran as an undercurrent and subtext to what I did daily?

The only relief I felt from the constant bombardment of self-perpetrated fat-hating was through dieting. When I was on a diet, I was doing the right thing. I was eating the right foods. I was on the "right" side. From the first day of the diet, my mood radically shifted. I was a part of the "them," the good. Even though my body looked otherwise from the outside, I knew this fat-suit was only temporary. In a few short months, I'd be on the other side! I'd blend in with all the other people who had it together.

When on a diet, I could take the imagined fat-hating from others because I knew I was changing, and the fat was melting away. I didn't blame "them" for not knowing I was in transformation. They were looking at the past, the old me. But soon, soon I would be thin because I was now good.

This idea was powerful. I couldn't sustain a diet, but the promise of being good from the moment I changed my eating habit – and I mean the moment I decided – brought me back to try again.

I didn't face a diet as a "try." Yoda was right! "Try not! Do or do not, there is no try." Almost every time I went on a diet, I believed I knew this was the one. The last one. Of course, it was the last one because I was good and not bad.

How could I go from living with this garbage in my mind for decades to being mostly clear of it, just a few cobwebs? The answer lies in much of the change I've talked about in this book. Deciding I was more interested in my mental health than what I was/wasn't eating and therefore addressing my mental health issues. But what I haven't talked about that I know is pivotal to my change is the effect of my husband's gift to me of unconditional love.

I wasn't going to talk about Christopher, because when I do I feel like I'm bragging. I understand people live in loveless marriages – or worse. I don't like to talk about the rich blessings I have of Christopher and our three children because I don't want people to feel bad. I'm just telling you how I feel, which I know is a projection that other people want what I want. Yes, yes, I know that not everyone wants a husband and three kids. But I do know everyone wants to be loved.

I wasn't going to talk about my luck in marrying Christopher because having the husband I have feels like winning the lottery. How can you tell someone to win the lottery?

I decided to write about Christopher because one major reason I was able to make peace with food was due to his unconditional love. He tells me - and I really believe him - he loves me. His love has not been different when I've been on a diet, off a diet, over 200 pounds, or close to my goal weight. There has been no discernable difference of love from him. Christopher is always on my side.

When I was sick with BED and depression, what did he do? Loved me. Helped me. Picked up my slack. Supported me.

That kind of unconditional love is a balm. My husband isn't perfect. We fight. He's disappointed me. I've disappointed him. Of course, this is the case. We've been married for 26 years.

Even in the hardest of rough patches, I never questioned his love for me.

If I was in a relationship where my partner made me feel bad for the state of my body or had the false belief that fat was bad … I have no idea where I'd be. Hopefully, out of the relationship. But I am keenly aware getting in and out of relationships, in particularly abusive ones, is difficult.

What I do know is that you are lovely and lovable. You are not loveable because of the size of your body. You have infinite value and worth. If there is no one in your life that loves you unconditionally, I'm very sorry. The good news is that you are not condemned to that state.

Love is amazing. When you love, love comes back. The more you love, the more you can give and receive love. The kind of love I am talking about here is not romantic love. It is the kind of love that is a decision. The decision to show up, be present, support, be interested in, and to serve.

If there is no one who loves you unconditionally, you might want to look at the people in your life and see if there is anyone who is a possible candidate. Have you closed yourself off to the love of others due to the hectic pace of modern life, family issues, past pain, food addiction, etc.?

We are social creatures by nature. We want to be loved. We are lovers. If you find yourself loveless, my best advice is to spend your time, attention, and creative energies growing your love-base. Love is magnetic. If you start to invest in others, you may be surprised what happens.

You may find it odd to bring up being loved in a book like this, especially when I tout your personal ability to change your situation. I feel like I'd be lying to you if I didn't tell you the truth of my transformation is in large part because of my support system. This life is hard. There is no reason to go it alone. We are here to help each other – really help each other. To love and be loved.

Being loved alone probably won't free you from food addiction, at least it didn't for me. But we'd all be fools to underestimate the power of love and being loved. Here is my very unscientific pie chart of what has helped me recover from BED:

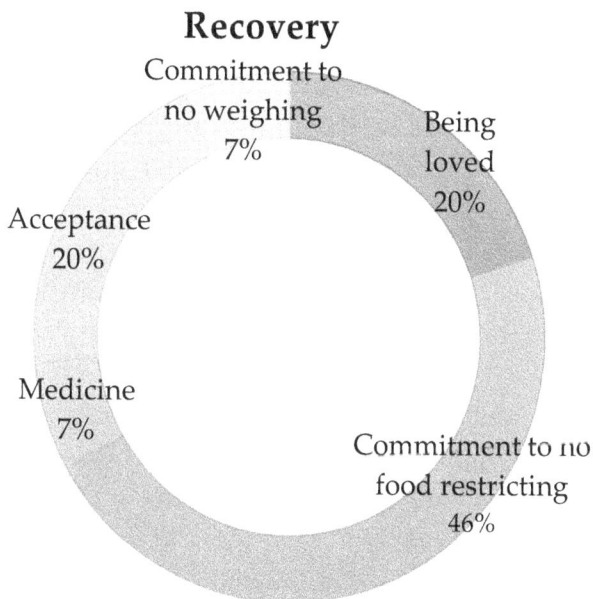

Recovery

Commitment to no weighing 7%

Being loved 20%

Acceptance 20%

Medicine 7%

Commitment to no food restricting 46%

Chapter 28: The Food Addict's Challenge

Can you imagine a life where you never diet again? Can you imagine a life where you make peace with food?

It's entirely possible!

How? How can you, if you are a food addict, become someone who isn't worrying about food and weight until the day you die?

Here are the two key steps you can take to achieve making peace with food.

Step 1: Understand what peace with food really is

Peace, for me, is not a state of living wherein I no longer have food issues. Peace with food is finding a way to co-exist with the addiction:

- Admit I have the addiction.
- Acknowledge it's not something that ever goes away.
- Decide to co-exist with the addiction.
- Manage the condition.

Peace with food is living in the present reality, not running away from the pain of the addiction. Whenever the negative food thoughts and/or behaviors appear, enlist your plan to deal with and not avoid the issue(s). My plan is simple, but effective for me.

I find peace with food in repeating my mantra: *You are not on a diet. You can eat anything you want.* I say it over and over, focusing on it instead of the voice that tells me I don't deserve to eat. Depending on the aggressiveness of the thought, I move on to repeating my mantra out loud with increasingly colorful language and volume.

I find peace with food by acknowledging when I have worrisome food thoughts. Instead of stuffing them down, I get curious about them. I resolve to observe the bad food thoughts and name them for what they are: thoughts passing through my mind. I am not those food thoughts.

I notice that somedays I am super hungry. I call these days "hungry days." I remind myself that not all days are "hungry days" and since I don't restrict - ever - I eat what I want on those days. When the anxious thoughts race, worrying, *"What if I will always feel this way? What if every day becomes a hungry day?"* I acknowledge that is a scary thought. I don't deny how I feel or the fear. Then, not discounting the worry, I parade through my mind my history and ratio of normal eating days and hungry days. I remind myself that I have a hungry day every few weeks. I remind myself this has been a regular pattern for years. I gently reason with myself that it is highly likely that today's hungry day will follow in a similar pattern. That is what will most likely happen. If it doesn't happen, and all my days turn to hungry days, I will deal with it. Either way, it will be okay.

Yesterday was a hungry day for me. I don't like them, but they are my reality. It's okay. Making peace with food is recognizing I have a condition that needs to be managed. Honestly, given where I am in recovery, most of my days in relation to food are fine. I'm telling you, I will go weeks without thinking about food. It's true. And yet, I still have hard days or even weeks. That's the reality. I am no longer shocked that I get assaulted by crazy food thoughts. This is part of the acceptance. This is part of the managing and healing: I am a food addict with a condition that must be managed. The management of the condition varies depending on what's going on in my life. This is how I've made peace with food. It's an imperfect peace, but a peace for which I am deeply grateful.[57]

---

[57] As I composed my list of how to make peace with food, I realize it could take some work. I know how to artificially inflate what I do. I

Step 2: Resolve to never diet again

I recognize this piece of advice is scary and may not work for everyone. Nonetheless, I encourage you to be open to the idea that your life of failed diets is not a result of your lack of willpower. Instead of self-beratement, discover your internal and external food addiction causes and triggers.

The next time you feel compelled to get back on a diet, consider trying the following instead:

- Determine the average length of the diets you've been on.
- Instead of food restricting, go on a fact-finding mission for that length of time.
  - Get curious about your food history.
  - Spend real time examining your internal and external food addiction causes and triggers.
  - Develop and fill out a pie chart of your relationship with food.
  - Seek the help you need. Depending on your issues, you may need help from some or all of the following:
    - Therapist
    - Trusted friend
    - Religious leader
    - Doctor
    - Nutritionist
    - Case worker
    - Attend Overeaters Anonymous

---

know what I'm supposed to say, that I have a list of people and a therapist to call, that I have an emergency contingency plan if I find myself in dire straits, but that would be false. I am still a work in progress. I need to work on my list of resources for when I'm facing food addiction troubles.

- Online support

The point of these months is to take your power back. Instead of being controlled by the vicious cycle of food addiction, **you** decide what you want in life. **You** decide what kind of life you want to live. **You** take an objective look at your food issues and the VARIOUS and creative ways **your** issues can be addressed.

Addressing rather than avoiding issues is the path to finding real solutions. As you go through this process, you may find your main problems are not what you think they are.

If you have a food addiction, I contend your main eating problems are not what you eat, but what you think about your body and food. Yes, even if you are hundreds of pounds overweight.[58] The battle of having a healthy body is fought and won in the mind. It is not fought merely externally by monitoring what is put into your mouth.

Sure, you could spend these months skipping this advice and do what you've always done. Restrict. But why? This is what you've done countless times before. Why not try something different? Why not try something novel and treat yourself – your entire self – with love, kindness, dignity, and worth?

The loving way to treat your body and mind is to get the help you need. You have a problem. Accept the fact that you

---

[58] Every person with an eating disorder, regardless of size, must learn to make peace with food. If you think someone is too overweight to take time to deal with the mental disorder, I wager you don't know what you're talking about. Sure, people can lose weight, but if we want mental health and the possibility of losing health-related weight, the mental must be addressed. Otherwise, you are dooming the person to the vicious cycle of yo-yo dieting, which is bad for the mind and the body. Let's stop treating people as objects to be controlled and instead as people to be loved.

have a problem and find the kind of support you need. Be creative. Be proactive. Be your own advocate instead of the imprisoner.

This path isn't easy. But neither is living in the hell of an out of control eating addiction. You've just got to pick your hard. If you decide to do something different and seek help, *HELP THAT IS NOT A WEIGHT LOSS PLAN, NOT A DIET*, you may find **your** path, what **YOU'VE** created, to make peace with food.

Where am I today, in the later summer of 2021? It amazes me, but I am finally at peace with food. I am mentally healthier in my relationship with food and my body than ever before. I continue to walk the tightrope of taking weight loss medicine to maintain my weight, while standing resolute that I will never diet (restrict) again. I am still working on incorporating exercise into my daily life. If writing this book has shown me anything, it's that we are all works in progress.

You deserve to be free from the tyranny of food addiction! You are so much more than what you decide to eat on any given day and the size and shape of your body. You are beautiful. I wish you all the luck in the world as you make peace with food.

The End

Acknowledgements

There are many people to thank for this book seeing the light of day. First and foremost, I am thankful for the extreme love, care, and support my husband has gifted me year after year.

I am thankful for Lisa Smartt, my decades long writing partner and friend.

Stephanie Richardson is the first person who sees my work and is unbelievably encouraging.

Sheila Scott graciously offered her incredible editing skills. I am thankful for her patience with me and diligent (and quick!) work.

I am incredibly thankful to my readers: Ashley Kite-Rowland, Alicia Field Pinto, Janet Manning, Robin Last, Nicolle Crist Gallagher, Jennifer Alexander, and Lexie Copeland.

I am very thankful for the excellent healthcare professionals in my corner; Elizabeth (Beth) Wade-Roberts, CRNP, and Michael Hinds, M.D. Beth listened to my situation, knew my past, and took the time to talk with me about my options in managing my eating disorder, including taking medicine. Dr. Hinds, my longtime family doctor, took my great falling apart seriously, caring for me through BED and clinical depression.

Lastly, a very sincere shout out to the awesome Martin, Tennessee coffee shops. The majority of this book was written as I bounced between Martin's Coffee and Bakery, Higher Ground, and Vantage. I am incredibly thankful for these awesome local businesses that provide not only excellent coffee and treats, but places for the community to gather, and in my case, write.

Appendix A: Religious Fasting Days

Since I have resolved not to restrict my food consumption, I deal with a reoccurring issue every year – religious fasting days.

For the first few years after I recovered from BED, and after much soul wrenching, I opted out from participating in fasting during Lent. I was not psychologically healthy enough to deal with it.

Since then, each Lenten season is a mixed bag. I always deal with whether I'm just copping out – coming up with an excuse to not have to do something hard. It's hard not to eat.

I come back to the truth of it. It's hard for me in a much different way than it is for most.

Some years, I don't have much of a problem. This year, 2021, was hard.

This year was hard because being on weight loss medicine has dredged up negative food thought patterns. For years, I thought not at all about what I was or wasn't eating. I utterly put an end to thinking about it or discussing it. So much freedom! Really! If you didn't spend puberty until the age of 30 something on a diet, it's hard to imagine the prison of every single day. Of talking to food. Of the cycle of utter disappointment and hatred of my body.

What is a fasting day like? For me, this year, it started as soon as I realized Lent was around the corner (about a month away). The conversation begins in my head.

Will I? Won't I? Should I? Am I still sick enough to not follow the rules? Am I well enough and just lazy and selfish?

This, played on a loop in the background, intensified as the day approached. Powerful self-scrutiny the days before. The day before the fast, I will have decided one way or the other - upset with my decision. But I know – it's all about the day. Can

I handle it? I usually convince myself, I just can't do it. I hate the crazy!

I've found, the way out for me is to not engage in the conversation. If I don't ask the question, I don't play the game. However, once the question is introduced, I get dragged in.

Will I fast?

What will I eat?

Can I opt out?

I had this problem on Ash Wednesday, but Good Friday was the worst. The lead up to Friday was intense. I had decided I needed to fast. But, when I woke up – it was a big fat no. I tried to fool myself at first, but I knew it was my decades old game of self-deception. I started with a coffee. I decided to take two of my boys shopping, an hour away. We went through the drive-thru at a local coffee shop and I ordered a mocha. I told myself, "Just a drink," but the game was already thrown. I wasn't going to follow the rules.

I half-assed it. I didn't snack in the afternoon, didn't have meat, but I did eat lunch and dinner. They were small meals, but I ate until I was full.

This was months ago, but thinking about it makes my skin crawl. My mind immediately goes to Lent 2022. What will I do then?

My default question needs to be, regardless of the situation, "Merry, how are you managing your addiction?" I think the wise decision is to put the question of fasting to rest, deciding not to fast until it is clear that I can without being thrown into the chaos of my abhorrent food mind. As I continue to heal, I have hope I will be able to fast at some point in my life.

Dealing with whether or not to fast is not a new question for me. The following is from a 3/16/2013 blog post I wrote about fasting:

You said you felt some anxiety toward the Lenten season – why is that? Have you found the deprivation/restriction period triggering?

ANY form of food restriction causes a chain reaction in my messed-up brain. If you tell me I can't have (fill in the blank), it's all I can think about.

Catholics fast (and this kind of fast actually doesn't mean no food all day) on the first day of Lent and Good Friday. I want to love God and follow the Church's teachings. Consequently, I do the mental gymnastics of trying to figure out if I'm doing well enough to participate in the fast or if I'm just trying to weasel out because I'm lazy. This year, thinking about whether I was going to fast on Ash Wednesday, and the accompanying anxiety, began at least three weeks before the date.

Have you come up with some safe ways to observe Lent without being at risk of relapse?

Yes. In the beginning, when I was sick, I searched the internet for advice and talked to my priest about my situation. He was really reassuring that fasting was only for those who were able and due to my condition, I was simply not able. He was right. Those first years I was unable to consider fasting.

Now, since I no longer have BED, I don't know what to do. A major contributing factor of my recovery is my commitment to never diet again. I don't count calories. I eat what I want. I do not restrict. I don't even know what I weigh!

So, how do I observe Lent? Right now, I'm taking it year by year. Honestly, this year I spent so much energy trying to figure out whether to fast on Ash Wednesday, I didn't give much thought to the rest of the forty days. Many people give up sweets, meat, soda, or something food related, but that's not necessary. Lent is a time to reflect on how much we need God's grace. The idea of giving something up, some very small sacrifice, is to point us toward God.

My best advice for someone with an eating disorder, who wants to participate in Lent, is to spend time reflecting on how great and vast God's love is, and to pray for healing.

Appendix B: Misunderstanding the Causes of Diet Failure

The following is an excerpt from my 2009 (thankfully unpublished) diet advice book. I am including this to show you I understand the argument and the desire to believe and promote the false idea that the only way to deal with overeating is by exerting self-control. I used to believe this too. I was wrong, but I saw no other way. I lacked imagination and only saw two options: restrict (be good) or be a glutton (be bad). What else is there?

But there is the third way. The third way realizes the way to treat a food addiction is by treating it as a physical and mental health issue. It is a reductionist lie to reduce and imprison the food addict to the **false narrative that follows**:

Blame, Blame, Blame. Blah, Blah, Blah.

Go ahead and blame the donut. Go ahead and blame the movie theater popcorn. Go ahead and blame the steak house steak, the fresh baked cookies, your mother, or your lover, your boss, your kids, or the universe.

What do you have to show for all your blame? What have you gained? I say you have gained a victim's mentality and your sense of courage, moderation, self-control, and overall sense of peace has been weakened.

Oh, but I feel better. I have something or someone to blame for my condition.

How absurd!

It's funny (and rather sad) to realize I have blamed so many external factors for my food obsession. I have blamed the way freshly baked bread smells, or the fact that brownies are too good not to be eaten. I have blamed the fact that I'm stressed out or that I've been a "good girl" and I deserve a treat.

Worst of all I've used the excuse that I am broken and there is nothing I can do about it, so why try? Believing that I could not resist. Believing that I did not have the ability to resist a Twinkie!?!

I am not a weak woman. I am a strong, independent, intelligent, funny, loving, kind woman … and a dessert addict. To look at myself from the point of view of all I have accomplished in my life and the fact that I truly like myself, it is unbelievable to me that I have allowed myself to be held captive and imprisoned by food.

My biggest excuse is that I have no willpower. Accept it and move on. This is just my lot in life. Who am I to fight fate?

This is your life. **Your one life**. How do you want to live it? Is your life truly yours? Do you hide from your choices and responsibilities?

I am not advocating for blaming the victim. Some have real and serious wounds due to the callousness of others. I am saying to choose a victim's mentality is to choose the life of oppression. Why give yourself up? Why allow wickedness to steal today from you and turn you into a shell of a person?

You are free. What are you going to do with your freedom? Are you going to let the past dictate what you choose to do today? Are you going to take-up the mess you've made and do something about it? Are you going to do the same-old, same-old and stay stuck?

The present is up to you. Your past and your future do not speak for you today. You choose who you are today. In fact, you are the sum total of your choices. Does this make you feel uncomfortable? It should.

The burden of human freedom is not to be taken lightly. You are the sum total of *your* choices. How you choose to deal with the everyday and the extraordinary are up to you. There is no written script for you. You are not an actor in a play that someone has already written. What you do today has not been chosen for you by God or the universe.

This is the burden: the realization that as a free being who I am is entirely up to me. What I make of myself and the events that occur in my life are on my shoulders.

I have been fighting eating issues since puberty. How I choose to deal with those desires and drives are exactly how I have chosen. Are there some unseen forces at work? Sure! I may be battling chemicals in my brain, and I am most certainly fighting some psychological issues. Yet it is I who decides to "give in" or get help. It is I who decides to take the easy way or stand firm in my resolve.

Since I've taken my food-life back from my passions I've been working on facing the damage I've done. I am trying to allow myself to mourn the loss of my beloved sweets. I am sad they are gone. I am sitting in my office right now and sad the vending machine in the basement is forever off limits to me.

It's okay to mourn. In fact, if you are being honest with yourself, you should mourn! I mourn no more funnel cakes! I mourn no more fried Snickers at the Reelfoot Craft Festival! I mourn no more Dairy Queen. Do not make light of the changes you are making. They are real and they are really painful. Painful!

I went into a homemade chocolate store with my friend, Laura. She purchased $16 worth of various fudges. I love fudge. Who doesn't? I inhaled trying to enjoy the smell for what it was. I knew I would not buy anything in the store. That self-knowledge made it easier to endure.

Laura and I were with a new friend. I turned to her and told her it would do me no good to get a little fudge, one chocolate dipped pretzel stick, or one of anything in the store because it would never be enough, never satisfy me.

Unfortunately, all she knows of me has been while I've been on this weight loss journey. I am admittedly too into food and calories at present – obsessed. And yet this is who I am at present. I know it is tiresome for those not on the journey to be with someone who has gone through an epiphany. I have hidden my unhealthy obsession with food for so long; I'm ready to be out in the open with my new commitment.

To be known is a frightful thing. To let someone in and see me, I find almost unbearable. And yet, I want to be known. I am trying to be honest with you, doing the best I know how.

***

This passage talks about freedom and finding help, but the only help I believed in was self-restraint. I was "free" because I was TIGHTLY in control of every single thing. I put in my mouth. My thoughts and conversations swirled around restricting food.

There is much I agree with in the above passage. This is your life. You do get to decide what to do. But your food addiction will not be solved through sheer self-determination. You need help. I thought taking stock of any cause or contributing factors to my lack of control were irrelevant and a hinderance to my goal: strict control of what went into my mouth.

I was as honest with myself as I could be. I saw no other way.

I decided to write this book because I wish I had known, long ago, that there are other ways to deal with food addiction.

Appendix C: 30 Days in the Life of a Food Addict

What follows is from the diary I kept when I was on my last diet. That diet spanned nearly one and a half years.

As you read this, I want you to keep in mind that I thought I was making good choices. I thought I was fighting the right battle (the battle of what I do or don't eat). At the time, I was proud of my constant restraint. In fact, I was in the middle of writing a book about freedom from food addiction through the virtues!

But now? Reading this brings me to tears. I'm so very sad for this person. I see the sickness ooze off the page.

The experiences and thoughts in this journal are not unique to my Last Diet Ever, except for being off sugar. Whenever I was on a diet, I would latch on to a few foods. Eating the same things were comforting. One less food decision to make.

You might find my focus on eating enough odd. My concern with eating enough on a diet comes from my Junior High School science teacher who convinced me that if you didn't eat enough, you'd end up like her – overweight even though eating under 500 calories. This has been a great fear I carried. (During this time, I didn't have a period for about 6 months. It was determined it was due to my diet. I wasn't eating enough.)

My pattern, as it is with most dieters, is restrict, restrict, restrict until the dam breaks. For twenty-five years I followed this pattern of plan to diet, diet (restrict), fall off the wagon. If you are not a food addict, I hope this diary gives you a glimpse of what some with food addictions deal with daily.

This is a peek into why I refuse to restrict. I will not bind myself like this again. I care too much about me. Thankfully, I've found a different way to deal with my addiction.

June 11, 2009

I went for a walk this morning; it was beautiful outside, but really humid. I had a SlimFast for breakfast. I love my SlimFast! While J and L were at Kid College this morning, T and I ran errands. Before we went to the grocery store, I stopped home for an apple and water. At the store, T got what we affectionately call chicken-balls from the deli. Of course, he wasn't interested in them, and I was left to wander the store slightly hungry with the scent of crunchy chicken within arm's reach, following me. I managed to make it out of the store without eating a single one! While shopping at the store I perused the cracker aisle in search of low(er) fat, low(er) calorie peanut butter crackers. I found some that were 180 calories a pack of 6 with 9 fat grams and 3 grams of fiber. In the car I opened a package for the baby who took a bite and, in diva fashion, threw the rest to the ground. I decided I wanted to *try* one too. Delicious. I decided, since it was 11a.m., to eat a package as a part of lunch. Halfway through the first package I began deliberating as to whether I could reasonably consume a second package as a part of my lunch too. I finished the first package (including the one the baby threw on the floor of the minivan) and decided to wait until I got into the house to figure out whether to have the second pack. Once I was able to pull myself away from the temptation and breathe fresh air, I said no (out loud) to seconds.

An hour later I sat down for (the rest of my) lunch: two servings of deli ham (a total of 2 points) and two slices of low-calorie bread. As a snack in my office, I drank a V-8. I've been having such problems in the evening with wanting to overeat. I told my husband to fix food just for him and the kids tonight. For some reason it feels easier to stay within my allotted calories for the day if I don't sit down at the table and take a portion of food, leaving the rest of the food staring at me. Chris fixed waffles for the boys and I went through the Taco Bell drive-thru for a bean burrito before I got home from work.

Chris is teaching a night class tonight and I decided to bake his students cookies. This goes against my rule of not baking treats, but I had two tubs of frozen cookie dough I bought from a kid I know. I baked one tub of cookies and brought them to Chris' students. It was hard being around the cookies, but not too terribly awful. After I dropped the cookies off, I told my husband not to return with any of them. When I went to clean up the kitchen, I noticed one lonely cookie had been left behind. I quickly threw it in the sink and doused it with water.

Tonight I didn't struggle with eating as much. Chris was at school teaching. The boys were in bed, and I relaxed on the couch reading. When Chris came home a little after 9 p.m., I realized I hadn't been thinking about food and not eating it for a while. A very nice change!

Today I weigh 140 pounds. I am down 55 pounds from where I started a little over a year ago. I have about 20-25 pounds I'd still like to lose, but my focus is (still) on wrestling my self-control back from my passions.

June 12, 2009
Walking this morning after the light rain was pleasant. I had a SlimFast for breakfast. For a snack at 10 a.m., I had an apple. Pink Lady apples are my favorites. Due to our summer schedule, Chris and I were able to eat lunch together. We walked to La Canasta and I had one fish taco without guacamole (even though they forgot and put it on, I successfully removed most of it). I figure the grilled fish taco has about 300 calories. Tonight, we went out of town with the boys to do a bit of shopping. I had my heart set on an extremely yummy veggie sandwich at Kirchoff's in Paducah, Kentucky. By the time we got to the deli, it was closed! We went to the restaurant next door instead. I ordered the salmon salad, sans the dressing. It was delicious, but not very filling. I had planned to eat a

large sandwich and even ate less yesterday, so it would fit into my calorie scheme. Once they finished eating, Chris took the boys to the car while I waited for the bill (you don't want to keep three young boys at a nice restaurant longer than necessary). As I waited, I calculated how many calories I had left, and I knew I needed to eat more. I had half a package of those peanut butter crackers in my purse and ate them. I also ate a small piece of bread from the breadbasket. It was a hard decision to end my calorie intake for the day there, in that way. I knew, however, if I didn't, I'd obsess about what I needed/should eat with the rest of my points until I did something about it. In the past I savored the idea of stretching out my eating as long as possible. These days I just want to get it over with and be done. Eating can be confusing! I had planned out my eating day, but food-life doesn't always go as planned. It's hard to go with the flow when it comes to food because you are dealing with extremely potent biological and psychological desires to eat!

June 13, 2009
I love Saturday! I slept in until 6:30 a.m. and took the baby for a walk around 7:30 a.m. It was a beautiful cool morning in my small town. I came home and had a SlimFast for breakfast. The family headed to the elementary school to play on the playground and stopped by the farmers market on the way home. Chris made his modified "North Italian Pasta" for lunch. He cooked the fresh white onions we had just purchased along with tomatoes and garlic in chicken broth, no oil. Instead of the prosciutto the recipe calls for, he used ham. He tossed in bow tie pasta, and we had a stellar lunch. Chris is a great, creative, and low-fat cook. He makes it so hard to not care about food! After lunch I went to the office to work and had an apple.

I was doing great today, until dinner time. Chris was serving at church tonight, so I decided to go to McDonald's, get food and head out to the park with the boys. I ordered my favorite grilled Southwestern chicken salad without chips, the sauce they put on the chicken, and salad dressing. They added chips. Oh well. I also ordered a yogurt parfait. This was a fine meal. The boys wanted me to go back to McDonald's for ice cream and I felt like obliging. The boys got plain vanilla ice cream and I got a yogurt parfait for the baby. As I was feeding T the yogurt, I could see what was happening to me. I knew he wasn't going to eat much of it, and I really wanted it. I tried to think of my own advice, tried to think about not giving in. I gave in I'm sad to say. I then went inside and ate a low-cal piece of bread. All and all I only went over my total calories for the day by 100 to 150. It is so hard to stay focused when temptation is around you. I've decided to add the yogurt parfait from McDonald's to my 'no' list for the foreseeable future!

June 14, 2009
I had my chocolate SlimFast for breakfast after my walk and an apple for mid-morning snack. For lunch, Chris took the older boys out and I stayed home with the baby. I had a Weight Watchers' frozen chicken dish; it was 5 points, 260 calories. For a mid-afternoon snack I had two pieces of low-calorie bread and a banana. Chris grilled pork for dinner and made side dishes of rice with spices and garbanzo bean and mixed vegetables. After dinner I was done eating. I lingered in the kitchen after cleaning up, counting my calories several times to see if I could eat more, but no, I was done. It was difficult to not eat anything more, but not so bad today – thank you God!

June 15, 2009

I got rained on this morning midway through my walk. Came home and had a SlimFast (am I boring or what?) for breakfast and an apple for a snack mid-morning. Chris and I met for lunch at La Canasta. I had what I always have there now, one grilled fish taco. Chris' Baja bowl looked so delicious. After I'd eaten my taco, I had to physically resist the urge of my arm to spear some of his excess cheese. I was feeling very anxious when I came home from work. My computer wasn't saving my book file and then it blue screened. I really freaked out. After I calmed down and worked out the problem, I reached for a V-8 out of stress (this is real progress for me. This kind of stress used to give me permission to go through the Dairy Queen drive-thru for a Reese's Peanut Butter Cup Blizzard with an extra topping of Butterfingers). For dinner Chris made his North Italian Pasta per my request. Since my anxiety was running high, I felt the need to stuff myself, so I heated a bag of frozen green beans and ate almost all of them. I then proceeded to eat two pieces of low-cal bread and half an apple. This did nothing to soothe my anxiety, leaving me to feel worse. By the end of the night, though, most of my anxiety had left.

June 16, 2009

I did not walk today. It's been a few weeks since I took a day off and my body has been telling me for a couple of days now to take a break. It's hard for me to believe that I have to *restrain* myself from exercising! I had a SlimFast for breakfast, an apple mid-morning and a turkey tomato sandwich for lunch. Mid-day I had blueberry Greek yogurt and for dinner Chris made a pork, rice, and veggie stir-fry. Delicious as always. After dinner I knew I had a few points left to eat and was deliberating as to whether I should be done for the day. Staring at me from across the kitchen was a package of peanut butter crackers. My husband suggested I eat ½ a package, which is only 2 points. I pontificated as to why I shouldn't because it will not satisfy me, and I will only want to eat the entire package plus when I'm done. Satisfied I was done eating for the day, but as soon as my husband left the kitchen I headed straight for the crackers. Yummy. As anticipated, after I ate my measly allotment of crackers, I wanted more. I thought about eating the rest of the package but decided not to. I left the kitchen and went about my evening business. I realized before I went to bed that after I left the kitchen I didn't think about food for the rest of the evening. Amazing!

June 17, 2009

It felt so good to go walking this morning. It was relatively cool for June. The sky was cloudy with chunks of dark pink and gold rays shooting through the western corner of my vision. Back at home I had a SlimFast. I had an apple for a snack and a bean burrito from Taco Bell for lunch. For a mid-afternoon snack I had a serving of cubed cheddar cheese and a few handfuls of carrots. Chris barbequed chicken for dinner. I cut my piece of chicken up and added it to a gorgeous salad overflowing with corn, black beans, carrots, green bell pepper, and mixed greens. No salad dressing; I've all but given up on salad dressing. Before the boys went to bed, they asked for ice cream. J usually gets his own, but tonight for some reason I was helping him out. I took the lid off the chocolate-chocolate chunk ice cream and was unexpectedly assaulted with its scent. Chocolate ice cream doesn't play around with its aroma – very strong and intoxicating. I didn't have any, and I wasn't badly tempted to have a bowl (or carton). I did promptly wash my hands clean of the ice cream that had gotten on them.

June 18, 2009

I had a SlimFast today after a lovely walk in the Tennessee humidity. I was hungry this morning and kept watching the clock to see if it was time for a snack. Around 10 a.m. I had an apple and a serving of deli turkey. For lunch I had a can of soup (Progresso pot roast) and a serving of whole wheat peanut butter crackers. It feels unnatural to restrict myself to one single serving! Chris had to teach class tonight which meant I was on dinner duty. As you can see, Chris has taken over the cooking responsibilities in our family. Cooking use to be rather evenly distributed between the two of us. Over the years it went from 40(me)/ 60(him) to 25/75 this past fall to 5/95 this spring. I currently couldn't be happier with this arrangement. I am still very mad at food and don't want to deal with the temptations that come with the cooking preparation. I realize what a luxury I have in my cooking husband. Someday he'll want me back in the kitchen, but until that day comes, I plan to participate as little as possible.

Before dinner, our family headed to a Kid College reception. Our two oldest boys were involved with a two-week summer camp at the university. The reception was to showcase what the students accomplished. I knew there would be a dessert tray. In the past they had a vast array of cookies but this year they had THREE sheet cakes in celebration of the program's 25th year anniversary. I was okay as I walked past the as of yet uncut cakes, but as I was leaving, the aroma of the much-desired wedding cake was everywhere. I was glad to leave. The cake smelled like an intoxicating poison.

Dinner was Taco Bell and McDonald's. Yes, I'm one of those moms who doesn't mind going through multiple drive-thrus. L got a happy meal, and I got a Southwestern chicken salad. J got a steak chalupa from Taco Bell. Once at Taco Bell, I suddenly realized I was more in the mood for a Bean Burrito. I ate the bean burrito and took the chicken off the salad and just ate the salad. You do know I'm mildly crazy ....

June 19, 2009

As I was walking this morning, I thought of those three luscious sheet cakes I encountered last night. I remembered how they smelled and wondered how I'd feel if I was left alone with one to eat as much as I wanted. For the first time, I felt hope. When I look into my cake-less future, I usually feel despair. When I think of being at one of my sons' weddings and not having cake I want to cry, usually. But today, I had hope that in 20 years or so I wouldn't even notice the cake and its appeal. Hope for my future that I might actually be healed.

Breakfast was the usual (SlimFast), followed by the usual (apple) snack at 10 a.m. I met my husband for lunch at La Canasta and had the usual there too (one fish taco). Around 4 p.m. I had a cup of Kashi cereal. Dinner was a simple affair consisting of cheese, bread, scoop of peanut butter, and a V-8 (I planned to have a V-8 but never got around to it. Instead, I went to my office after dinner and consumed an entire pack of spearmint gum – 18 pieces! This is not the first time, so I think it means no more gum for me in the near future).

June 20, 2009

Breakfast: SlimFast
Snack: Apple
Lunch: chicken noodle soup
Snack: Another apple and a few handfuls of grapes.

My friend had a birthday party for two of her children today at the university pool. I knew cupcakes would be there waiting for me. Though I wanted one, I honestly wasn't desperate to eat one. Laura is good about food. Her party consisted of a variety of baked potato chips, grapes, apples, and juice boxes. And the cupcakes. Pretty healthy fare for a kids party.

I was trying to eat light during the day in anticipation of the date night my husband and I had planned. We went to the Opera House where I had the salmon on rice with a side of broccoli and a garden salad. This was a fine meal that fit within the remainder of the calories I had left for the day. I told myself ahead of time that I would not have a roll with dinner. And then the basket of rolls came. My husband took one without thinking about it and ate it. I knew it was soft and sweet, probably warm too. I was able to neglect the bread while eating my dinner, but once I was done the bread started shouting at me. Why is eating so hard? I am tired of constantly fighting, always counting what I'm eating, being aware of food. I was feeling okay about food the past few days, but not today. Why can't I be done with food? I wish I didn't care what it tastes like. Maybe I really shouldn't care. I don't know how not to care. After dinner we went to a coffee shop. He got coffee and a warmed cinnamon bun, and I bought water and a cup of fresh fruit. His roll was topped with a distracting amount of frosting. To make matters worse, after the coffee shop we went to the movies. The smell of the movie theater popcorn was gripping. I dealt with it.

I feel like I'm hanging on, barely. I could fall off into oblivion again, but I *really* don't want to. I feel like I'm finding myself and I don't want to lose me.

Food, food, food. When will I be done with my love of food?

June 21, 2009

I was not looking forward to today. Father's Day means lots of food everywhere, all day long.

After my walk I made breakfast for the family: muffins and egg sandwiches. I then drank my SlimFast. I didn't find it difficult to cook for them and not eat it. Being Father's Day, I decided to oversee the babies at church. For most of the mass T and I hung out in the social hall, where I inhaled the scent of cooking sausages for nearly an hour. The smell wasn't too bad, and I found myself pausing several times to enjoy the smell of the delicious food I would not consume. After church I battled the spread. It was only the glazed donuts that taunted me. After mass I dropped Chris, J, and L off at home and went to the grocery store with T. It was 10:30 a.m. by this time and I was ready for a snack, but for some reason I can't remember I didn't take the time to go in the house and get an apple. Big mistake. It is eating healthy 101 to not enter a grocery store hungry! As per usual, I started off at the bakery to get the baby chicken balls. We headed to the back of the store, and I literally started salivating as my internal battle raged as to whether or not I could have just one chicken ball. Somehow, I made it home without eating anything but one grape. As soon as I got home, I had 10 minutes to get J, L, and myself ready for a birthday party potluck at the park. I was really dreading this. Not the people or the party, of course, but the food. I decided yesterday to eat my lunch today before I got to the party, this way I didn't have to make any food decisions – I would eat nothing. I wolfed down a ham tomato sandwich and a cup of Kashi cereal. This is the first day of summer and boy it sure was! It was so hot at the park, we only lasted an hour. Turns out my food worries were unfounded because they hadn't even started eating by the time we left. I came home and had an apple. After an all too brief nap, I had 2 servings of grapes and a piece of bread. I hadn't planned on any afternoon snack, let alone three, because we were going out to dinner to celebrate Father's Day. Isn't this sad? It's Father's Day, a day to celebrate what an excellent dad Chris is, and I am focused on myself and food, not on him.

Eating out is full of peril! I had planned to get a grilled chicken salad at the Mexican restaurant Chris chose, but guess what – they didn't have one. I know, unbelievable! All their salads were in fried shells with lots of goop in them

(I think goop is cheese, sour cream, guacamole, beans, and oil). Chris found something rather inoffensive for me to eat, the wheat quesadilla, filled with grilled veggies and choice of meat. I chose shrimp (even though I really wanted the chicken, but figured the calories saved would help to offset the cheese that was sure to be in the quesadilla). My meal came, sans sour cream, and my eyes bulged. It was huge! I immediately divided it in half. I decided to just trash most of the wheat tortilla instead and eat the insides. It was filled with yummy grilled vegetables and shrimp, but there was cheese and oil too. By the end of dinner, I felt like a loser because I ate all the guts and half of the tortilla, *and* half of my son's flour tortilla. Once I start eating it is so hard to stop. Like a shark. What should I have done? Ordered something different, or better yet, waited to eat until I got home.

My torture continued tonight as I made the boys a bedtime snack of peanut butter and jelly sandwiches. I wanted just one scoop of peanut butter, or a yogurt that was sitting by the jelly. I wanted but didn't eat and was still disappointed with what I ate at dinner. What can I do now? I have the opportunity to practice the virtue of compassion and kindness directed at myself.

June 22, 2009

I was hoping to eat lightly to make up for my quesadilla sins last night. All went well until dinner time. After I ate my sandwich and cheese, I planned to wait to have a cup of Kashi cereal. I reminded myself I'm trying not to drag out mealtimes anymore, so I should get it over with ASAP. So, I had a cup of Kashi, and then another 1/3, and then another 1/3, and then a final 1/3. I was immediately mad at myself, kicking myself for not stopping. If I eat until I am full, or more than my reason tells me to eat prior to the commencement of eating, I am out of control. Well, if I eat more than I intend to then I'm not in total control.

Someday, someday in my near future my head will take full control of what I eat. I feel much more hopeful today.

I felt so full after eating all that fiber rich cereal (10 g per serving) and I felt bad. When I'm full, regardless of what I've eaten, I feel like I've done something wrong. I knew, even with consuming that extra serving of cereal, I was still within my points of the day. I've been counting points so long I wondered what my food day looked like if I just looked at the calories. This was what I ate today:

Breakfast: SlimFast 230 (4)
Snack: Apple 80 (1)
Lunch: Soup 140 (2)
        Yogurt 80 (2)
Dinner: Cheese 120 (3)
        Ham 45 (1)
        2 cups cereal 280 (4)
        Bread, 2 slices 80 (1)
        Tomatoes, 40 (0)
Total: 1195, 19 points

June 23, 2009
After a lovely walk, I had a SlimFast. I took the boys to the local pool in the morning and came home and ate an apple. For lunch I ate turkey and lettuce roll-ups, tomatoes, yogurt, and one spoonful of peanut butter. I was full after lunch and immediately started to feel regret for eating so much. I told myself over and over that though I ate a lot, all the foods and quantities were fine – lunch was a total of only 5.5 points. We invited some friends over for dinner and I was dreading the food choices before me. Since it was a spur of the moment invite, the menu for dinner was Domino's pizza, watermelon, salad, lemonade, and ice cream. I was worried about eating the pizza. How much should I have? Could I really have two pieces, or should I strictly stick with one? I had one piece of cheese pizza, several helpings of salad and half a watermelon. As I was putting the leftover

pizza in the refrigerator, I ate three corners of the thin crust pizza Chris ordered. Ugh!

After dinner and a fun theological conversation, Chris and D. took the boys outside for a game of baseball. A. and I stayed inside and chatted. I noticed (I'm ashamed to admit) A. ate only one piece of pizza too, and it turns out she is on Weight Watchers also. We talked about weight issues and our own craziness. I mustered the courage to tell her I am writing a book about my own issues. She was very sweet and encouraging. I really want to tell all my friends and family and strangers walking down the street what I'm up to. But I don't … not sure why.

June 24, 2009
SlimFast for breakfast and an apple for snack. I watched the clock for the apple snack from 8:30 a.m. until time to eat.

Lunch was veggie soup, 2 servings of deli sliced chicken, ½ cup Kashi cereal, and two pieces of low-calorie bread. After my seminar, I had a V-8. I don't think I've mentioned this before, but every day, throughout the day, I drink water. I shoot for 64 ounces of water a day and usually hit the mark.

At dinner, I achieved a small feat I am proud of. Chris decided to spend the early evening mowing, so I took the kids to the next town over to run errands. For dinner we ended up at Taco Bell. I had not eaten much today and still had about ½ of my points remaining. I usually get a bean burrito at Taco Bell, which is 6 points. What to do with the four remaining? I could string out the eating experience, but I'm working on eating and getting it over with. I decided to order 2 bean burritos, cutting the second one in half. As soon as I sat down with the food, I divided the second burrito and offered it to the boys. They nibbled on it but were not interested. By the time I consumed my allotted 1 ½ burritos I began eyeing the remaining half. Would it be so bad to just eat it? It's only three points. I'm still hungry and it looks so good. Maybe just a bite of the tortilla … No. I stopped my thoughts, wrapped the burrito up and put it on the other side of the table with the trash. A victory for me! Every time I am able to resist my lusts, I grow stronger. Maybe there will come a time when I don't even consider eating the other half, not even tempted. Regardless, I will continue to fight my immoderate desires.

Once the kids went to bed, Chris and I sat down to watch a movie. I was considering eating a bag of frozen vegetables and decided to eat it. On Weight Watchers most vegetables don't count for points. They're free. But I wondered, what does this say about me if I choose to eat 4 servings of vegetables? Is this immoderate? (As it turns out, I found out later, 4 servings of veggies do count toward the total points for the day!)

June 25, 2009
A lovely walk, as usual. Unusually, however, after I drank my SlimFast I was hungry within half an hour. A SlimFast staves off my hunger for about 3 hours. Wonder why today is different? For a snack I had grapefruit – delicious! I had plans with Laura and Diane for a late lunch. A late lunch today? I was ready for my second meal at 10 a.m. I took the boys to the public pool and afterwards decided to have a light second snack to tide me over until 1 p.m. It started with one serving of deli chicken, which turned into 2 servings, and then I ate an entire bag of frozen veggies. Technically I only ate 2 points worth of food. As I mentioned yesterday, (I thought) most veggies don't count in your points total. But I had 4 servings and each serving is 70 calories. Each serving of meat is 1 point. But my total calories between the meat and vegetables was 380 calories! I decided to count the veggies as 3 points. So, even before I went to

lunch with my friends, I'd eaten 10 points! We were trying out a new restaurant in town (an old restaurant that reopened) and I wasn't sure what I could get for around 5 points (approximately 250 calories). Chicken veggie salad? On the way there Laura read an article in our local paper that boasted of its salad bar – great, I thought … I ordered the salad bar and went through the line. It wasn't as fresh as claimed in the paper. I did have a bowl of grapes and strawberries, and I did only eat about 3 points worth of food, two big pluses in my book. Draw backs – both Laura and Diane ordered the Gyro with fries. Their food looked delicious. After lunch we went to a matinee. You know what that means – the amazing, comforting smell of theater popcorn. Luckily, we were running late and consequently there was no time to stare longingly at the treats I would not buy. By the time I got home I was starving, and the sweet smell of chicken curry was everywhere. I had to wait a long 30 minutes until the chicken was ready. I wanted to know precisely how many points in a serving, but Chris was running late, and I was too hungry to figure it out. I ate a serving, with a ½ cup of rice. I am ashamed to say I went back for seconds, sans rice. When dinner was over, I was struck with the paradox. I still wanted to eat, wanted more chicken, more curry, maybe a yogurt. I was also feeling too full and therefore guilty. How can I, at the same time, feel shame and defeat for eating too much and the overwhelming desire to eat more? I was alone in the kitchen when I started to clean up. I said, out loud, "I am done eating for the day." I then turned these words into the following silly, yet effective, song, determined to sing it until I believed it: "I am done, I am done, I am done eating for the night." I ended up singing it over a hundred times, about the time the kitchen was clean. I sang it and towards the end of my sorry little song, I started to believe it – that I really was done eating for the day. I sang it again as I made J an after-dinner snack. I sang it again later as L requested more to eat, and once again as my baby uncharacteristically went to his highchair at seven o'clock at night – his bedtime - and said "eat" as he attempted to scale it. It is good to be done, to not have to fret over any more food choices for the day.

June 26, 2009

I thought today would be a relatively easy food-choice day … it seems like every day is an exception to the rule. Back from my walk I had a SlimFast. I was hungry, again, sooner than usual and was out of fruit. For a snack, I had a can of vegetable soup. Around 11:30 a.m., I was back in the kitchen. This time I ate two slices of low-calorie bread. Chris wanted to go out to lunch, a later lunch (anything past noon is later) and I have a hard time saying no to him. We met for lunch, J and L in tow. I ordered ONE fish taco and they brought me two! Ugh! Chris echoed the devil on my shoulder and said I should just eat them both. "No," I snapped. Chris shrugged and began eating my extra one. Halfway through he put it down and began on his own lunch. I looked at my little fish taco and wondered if it really was 300 calories/6 points as I estimated. Maybe I could eat mine and the extra half and call it 8 points? I took his half before I'd even finished my own. I consumed more than planned and was nowhere near full. The problem of eating a lot by 1 p.m. today was tonight we had plans to attend a university banquet. I knew there would be a salad. The yummy bread roll I'd been thinking about was now off limits. Around 3 o'clock I was back in the kitchen, this time eating TWO yogurts. I now had roughly 4 points/200 calories left in the day to eat. Going over, making an exception for myself today was not an option. At the banquet I had a large green salad, mixed steamed vegetables, and a breadstick I blotted over and over again. After dinner, Chris and I drove down to our favorite coffee shop where I ordered a cup of fruit. Thus ended my day of weird eating.

June 27, 2009

Today will be a normal eating day, right? We decided to go to Paducah, so the kids could play at Ya Ya's Island, and I could do some shopping. We would get in town just in time for lunch. Chris wanted to go to the excellent deli, and I did too – a little too much. With all the eating out I've been doing as of late, I decided on my walk this morning to bring my own lunch and not eat at the deli. I really wanted the hummus veggie sandwich but knew it would be better for my self-control to have a victory rather than my stomach. On the way to Paducah, I ate an apple and drank my water. Once there I ate 2 cups of Kashi cereal while Chris had a pork tenderloin sandwich and two cookies from the bakery. I dropped the kids and Chris off at the play place and went shopping. First off was a bathing suit. Never had I looked forward to this kind of shopping. Today, however, I was not filled with fear and trepidation. I went right up to the swimsuits, picked out a few to try on, and found just what I was looking for. Never before in my entire life have I looked in a mirror with a bathing suit on and felt I looked good. What a strange and wonderful feeling. After I finished my shopping, I picked up the family and we all headed to the bookstore. Ready to check out, I went to the café for water. They had water, along with many delights. I scrutinized the litany of bad choices, trying to find *one* item I could eat. Teriyaki beef jerky. I bought water and beef jerky! The jerky was only 80 calories for the entire pack. On the ride home I ate the jerky, another apple, and a V-8. Chris was serving at church tonight, so I made a simple meal for the kids, and I ate a serving of deli chicken, 2 pieces of low-calorie bread, a bag of mixed veggies and vanilla yogurt. As I cleaned, I began to sing my song, proclaiming to myself, until I believed it, that I was done eating for the night.

June 28, 2009

I decided not to walk this morning; I've been having foot issues since last fall. It is incredibly frustrating to want to exercise and have your body, a tiny part of your body, not cooperate. I've been thinking about seeing a physical therapist. Chris made waffles for the boys, and I had a SlimFast. After Mass I took T to Jackson (about an hour south) to do more shopping. I went back and forth in my mind as to what to do about lunch and decided to pack my own. On the way to Jackson, I ate an apple. The entire trip I wanted to eat, desperately wanted something in my mouth. It was a strange realization to reflect on not being hungry and still wanting to eat. I kept on checking the clock to see when I could eat my lunch. I had planned to shop before I broke into the food, but I was lucky to make it to Jackson (11:30 a.m.) without pulling over to eat. Lunch consisted of two pieces of low-calorie bread, 7 cubes of cheddar cheese (120 calories) and two servings of deli meat (100 calories). I then proceeded to shop. I had the wonderful problem of choice! Almost everything I tried on I liked on *me*; it was surreal. Most items I had to try on in smaller sizes. 3 ½ hours later, T and I made our last stop at Sam's club. I was hungry now and it was hard to ignore all the free samples. I gave most of the samples to T, save the slice of ham. Once we got to the car I drank my snack of V-8 and the bottle of water I bought. Chris made a delicious dinner, as always, of BBQ pork loin, rice, veggies, and I brought home watermelon and cherries. I weighed out and ate one 3 oz serving of pork, a spoon full of rice, half the vegetable medley and half of a watermelon. It was a hard day, a day when I wanted to eat all day long and so much looked and smelled good to me. I felt focused on my goal of being in control of what I ate and when I ate it. A good feeling, self-control – though it still is not without a sting for me, for I still cannot tell what will win in the end, my desire to be in control or my desire to eat whatever I want, when I want it.

June 29, 2009

It was a cool 60 degrees this June morning. It was good to be out on a walk. I really missed being out yesterday. I came home and made the boys lemon poppy seed muffins while I drank a SlimFast. Today will be another out of the norm eating day because I have a lunch date with my friend Michelle and dinner with my friend Weslee. After breakfast we lazed around with the boys jumping on the bed, wanting me to read to them. I had barely begun before the first kid was off to the kitchen for snacks. 10 minutes later with many snacks on my bed, we resumed. I had to endure the smell and crunch of sour cream and onion Pringles. I was happy to be done reading around 10 a.m. when it was time for my apple snack. I had a nice lunch with Michelle and ordered my usual fish taco. By 2 p.m. I was hungry again and drank a V-8. Soon after I came home, around 3:30, I ate the rest of the watermelon I cut up the night before. L ate a bit of it, and I ate the rest. This was not in my food plan for the day but decided to let myself eat it anyway (I'm still uncertain if I should have let myself). Dinner with Weslee was great. We went to Applebee's in the next town over. What an absolute delight to choose a meal from a menu offering several meals with Weight Watchers' points figured. I chose the Cajun tilapia and was not disappointed. After dinner we went to my favorite coffee shop to chat some more. I chose the fruit cup and water. I dropped Weslee off at her house and stopped off at Wal-Mart before heading home. Shortly after wandering through Wal-Mart, I realized I was hungry and ready to eat. I started to softly sing my "done for the night" song and it helped the longing. All and all a fine eating day, though I think I over did it on the fruit. On a scale of 1 to 10, 1 being a breeze and 10 being in the pit of despair with me being on fire, I'd give today a 5. I tell you, the shear monotony of abstaining hour after hour is not for the faint at heart!

June 30, 2009

Another lovely morning in Martin. Once home, I drank a SlimFast and was hungry within the hour. Ugh - not again … I ate an apple earlier than usual and drank a large glass of water that really helped with the hunger. I took the boys swimming and later to Taco Bell for them and the McDonald's drive-thru for me. Yes, I am a grown woman and I willingly go to McDonald's (for their Southwestern grilled chicken salad, without chips, sauce on the chicken, and salad dressing). Since the salad the way I eat it has only four points, I came home and ate a vanilla Fiber One yogurt and fought (and won) with a grapefruit who apparently didn't want to be eaten. I was still hungry. A little while later, I had 1 ½ cups of Kashi cereal and a glass of water. A few hours later, I had a V-8. I'd eaten a lot, but had left myself 4 points, enough to have a 3 oz serving of the salmon Chris was grilling for dinner, along with the green salad, and side of corn he prepared. We sat down at the table as he pulled the salmon from the grill. It was then that he mentioned the fish smelled very fishy before he put it on the fire. He was going to be the guinea pig. He didn't even take a whole bite before he was spitting it back out – rotten fish. We loaded the kids in the car and went through the Taco Bell drive-thru (yes, my kids had the same Taco Bell meal for lunch and dinner … not good). My bean burrito had 6 points, which I ate, along with a huge salad and serving of corn. I ate more than I'd anticipated for this day. I am working on the virtue of compassion today. I could have had more self-control mid-day with my snacks, and I could have cut 1/3 of my burrito off. I could have and did not. What worries me is I felt compelled to eat – and I enjoyed it, though the pleasure was over way too soon. I'm working on accepting less than perfect days.

I've been thinking about starting some kind of eaters group. At the public pool this morning, I saw two of my friends I wanted in the group. I casually mentioned it to them, and they were both excited to get together and talk about eating issues. By the time we left the pool, the first meeting of the Existential Eaters Society (EES) was planned for tonight, my house, 7:30 p.m. I came home and called two other friends I thought would be interested, and by luck or providence they were interested and available. We had a great time. We spent two hours talking about our journeys, admitting our craziness, and encouraging one another. We planned to meet again next week.

July 1, 2009

My foot has been bothering me again, but after stretching it out this morning I decided to go on a walk anyway. I came home and had my usual breakfast. Eating breakfast is important to me. I don't eat when I first get up, but usually 1 ½ to 2 hours later. I have noticed lately I've been hungry within an hour of having my SlimFast – I just must endure I suppose. Lunch was a salad, a bag of mixed veggies, 1 ½ scoops of peanut butter, two pieces of low-calorie bread and a Fiber One vanilla yogurt. And then … disaster! Within two hours of eating lunch, I had four or five more scoops of peanut butter and 1 ½ servings of cereal. By 1:45 p.m. I had eaten all my allotted points/calories for the day!

I really don't know what to say. I am utterly disappointed with myself, mildly devastated. Where was my role model? Why didn't I just stop? Will I ever be healed? Will I live forever on the edge of the precipice, not knowing moment to moment whether I'll jump? I am so messed up, so broken. What alternatives do I have? I could get up from my computer and raid the office snack machines? Make a run for a Big Mac and supersized fries? I know, I KNOW I don't want that life. I don't want to be out of control ... I am back to fervently wishing to never eat again. I hate you, stupid food! Some days it feels too hard, too much to ask to turn my back on nature. Not a stellar way to bring in the new month.

After my afternoon failure, I went to the office and cried. I worked a bit but was emotionally spent. Chris agreed to watch the kids, so I could be by myself and see a movie. The movie was mind numbing and did the trick. Once out of the theater I started crying again. I am so disappointed in myself. It is hard to be human, fallible, and fragile. The peanut butter debacle is over. I choose to no longer dwell on this failure, and instead to see it as a wake-up call, showing me I must remain vigilant. I am, however, going to cool it on peanut butter and Kashi cereal for a week or so. And in case you're wondering, I didn't eat anything more after 1:45 p.m. this afternoon.

On a happier note, I weighed myself this morning: 136.6 pounds.

July 2, 2009

Last night, I dreamt I ate a chocolate bar. I was repulsed and shocked by my actions in the dream. This must be leftover guilt and shock from yesterday. I had a sobering walk this morning. Still mad at myself, I thought about my husband's encouraging words last night. What was I to learn from my lapse yesterday? How could I make friends, or at least peace with food? The virtue that came to mind this morning was courage. The courage to keep on eating. The coward in me wants to overreact to yesterday's binge by seriously reducing my food consumption to a trickle – I'm not sure I'm capable of such depravation. Today, I'm going to think of courage.

After my walk, I had a SlimFast and an apple later for a snack. Lunch consisted of another SlimFast (obviously still mad at myself). Mid-day snack was a V-8 and dinner was

Chris' yummy North Italian Pasta. I didn't want to eat anymore after dinner, but since I had three points left for the day, I felt I should. I decided on a granola bar, the kind with 2 per package. One and a half bars equal three points. I opted for one bar. After eating it I decided to have the ½ too. My husband handed it to me and said, "And that's all you get to eat for the day." I was shocked! In the 15 years I've known him, he has never once said anything about my eating, never even hinting. I immediately put the half granola bar down, having lost my appetite. He saw immediately what he did given my reaction and started apologizing. He was just trying to help me, but I made it clear that kind of help sends me to the closet to eat by myself.

July 3, 2009

Another beautiful July morning. I don't know what's wrong, but it was cool this morning – in Tennessee in July! After drinking my SlimFast, I was off to the office to work. I still feel flat (the best word I can think of) about eating. How can food give life and be toxic too?

Mid-morning snack was an apple. I knew we were going out to dinner tonight, so I had a light lunch of two slices of low-cal bread, two servings of turkey lunch meat, and a yogurt. I had a V-8 for a mid-afternoon snack. I saved enough points to have two fish tacos at La Canasta but couldn't make up my mind as to whether I should eat two or save my points for something else later. After a few hours of vacillating back and forth, I still hadn't made up my mind when it came time to order. I automatically ordered one and that was that. After I ate one, I proceeded to eat a few bites of L's rice and ¼ of his flour tortilla. The family drove to the coffee shop in Union City for treats, where I had a cup of fresh fruit. While I bathed the boys, I ate a bag of steamed vegetables. I'm not entirely sure if I ate enough today, but close enough. The uncertainty had me in the kitchen, looking around for something more. I began to sing my song ... I am done, I am done, I am done eating for the night. The kids went to bed and Chris and I decided to watch *Pride and Prejudice*, the one with Colin Firth as Mr. Darcy. Taking a break mid-way through, I decided to get a bit more to eat – ½ cup of Kashi cereal. Much to my surprise, I made peace with this decision almost immediately.

July 4, 2009

We took a family walk this 4th of July morning. When home, Chris made pancakes for the boys, and I had a SlimFast. I had an apple for a mid-morning snack. For lunch I had two garden burgers, two pieces of low-calorie bread, and vanilla yogurt. Around 2 p.m., I had a V-8 and later a serving of beef jerky. For dinner, Chris grilled hamburgers for the boys and a bean burger for me. I had the spicy black bean patty, 1 serving of cheddar cheese, tomatoes, and lots of watermelon. After dinner Chris took the two older boys to a fireworks show and I ate a steamed bag of vegetables.

I wasn't supposed to weigh today, but my husband always weighs on Saturday mornings, so the scale was in the bathroom. 134.6 pounds – that's exactly 60 pounds. I'm very pleased!

July 5, 2009

I enjoyed my walk this morning. It was cool and humid, which made me sweat a lot. I always prefer to come home from exercising sweaty – makes me feel I worked hard. I had a SlimFast for breakfast and apple for snack. The family went to Los Portales for lunch today. I knew I would order the chicken salad, which consists of lettuce, tomato, green bell pepper, shredded cheese, and grilled chicken. Doesn't sound too bad, until you see it – it's huge. Ahead of time I decided to eat the whole thing, figuring it's about 500 calories/10 points. I had decided to eat the whole thing ... then it came. Psychologically it was difficult to be okay with eating such a massive salad, but I ate it, nonetheless. In the afternoon, I drank a V-8. We decided to order pizza for dinner, cheese for the boys and bacon/ranch for Christopher. I was resolved not to eat pizza tonight due to the large lunch I consumed. I had two servings of Kashi cereal and a grapefruit instead. As I was cleaning T's tray, the pizza was calling to me, saying, "... just one bite? Come on, finish me off. What will one little square of pizza hurt?" I answered (in my head) a resounding no. This was an opportunity to be courageous and stare down my appetites, an opportunity for my self-control to grow. I won the battle of the pizza tonight. Once the kids were in bed, I popped a bag of frozen vegetables in the microwave and ate them while Chris had his usual nighttime ice cream.

July 6, 2009

As I walked around the university track this morning, I thought of the pizza last night and smiled. I did it. I am gaining self-control. Pizza, for me, is a food I am learning to eat moderately. I am unwilling, however, to give into the temptation to eat something caloric, like pizza, after having a large lunch. For breakfast and morning snack, I had the usual. The kids started swim lessons today. Immediately after swim lessons we packed up the family and headed to Trappist, Kentucky where Chris was going on a spiritual retreat for the week. I packed my own lunch and ate it on the way: two pieces of bread, two servings of lunch meat, yogurt, and another apple. I packed a variety of treats to keep the boys occupied. The one's that tempted me? Animal crackers, chocolate teddy grahams, and shortbread cookies. After lunch I wasn't hungry, but really wanted to eat. There is something about being in a car that makes me want to put food in my mouth. Into the trip I had the carrots I packed, and Chris had the shortbread cookies, which I opened for him and deeply inhaled the aroma (they smelled much better than I anticipated). Four hours later we arrived and said goodbye to Chris. I had a V-8 to tide me over until we found a Subway. I had a foot-long veggie sub. Why a foot-long? I had 10 points/500 calories left and didn't want to prolong my eating. When I got back in the car I was stuffed. The only thing I consumed on my way home was lots of water.

July 7, 2009

Chris is gone for the week, so how am I going to exercise? I've been turning this over in my head for months, trying to figure out the best solution. I could dust off my old aerobic videos, I could walk around the back yard for an hour, I could pay a babysitter to come over in the morning for an hour. Our summer babysitter, AnnMarie, has agreed to come over this week before she goes to work.

Today, I had a SlimFast for breakfast, an apple for a mid-morning snack, a McDonald's grilled Southwest chicken salad for lunch, beef jerky in the afternoon, and 2 eggs, 2 spicy black bean patties, and a bag of steamed vegetables for dinner.

This afternoon was a torturous reminder of the power of the smell of food. First, it was the perfectly fried McDonald's French fries my son ordered. Next, it came blow-by-blow as I opened individually wrapped Snickers bites in the movie theater for said son. And after the movie we walked through the lobby in the middle of fresh buttery popcorn being popped. The smells were quite gratuitous! I know how delicious these foods taste. Why parade this fact under my nose? Tonight, after dinner, I was semi-full but very unsatisfied. I wanted to eat more, eat something sweet, anything really. Is it because I'm missing my husband? Am I bored? I don't know why, but it feels like I'm pulling my teeth out to keep from putting anything other than water in my mouth tonight.

July 8, 2009

My eating day did not go as planned. I was going to eat lightly today and take the boys to Applebee's for dinner. I had a late breakfast of SlimFast and apple, shortly thereafter. By the time I got to lunch, I felt really hungry – more than usual. I had a serving of cheddar cheese and a Weight Watchers' frozen meal of shrimp and pasta. I then decided to add a cup of my favorite Kashi cereal. A bit later, I had another apple and an hour later, a V-8. Since I'd eaten more than planned, Applebee's was now out. I ate dinner early, which consisted of 2 cups of Kashi cereal, a bag of frozen veggies and ½ a serving of cheese. I had such a hungry day. When I ate up all my points, I was still hungry. I started singing my "I am done" song, which helped a little. Why can't I just eat more … just one cup of delicious Honey Bunches of Oats with ice cold milk or the peanut butter crackers my kids snacked on all day? I don't know why I was (am) so hungry today. I just have to endure it, live with the pain and misery of not getting what I want.

July 9, 2009

I woke up early this morning to work, around 5 a.m. I don't like to eat before I walk in the morning, which is not typically an issue, but with my husband gone I had to wait until 7:30 a.m. to walk, which meant breakfast wasn't going to happen until 9 a.m. I was hungry almost right away but decided to wait. If I ate (drank) breakfast by 6 a.m., lunch would take forever to arrive! I made it until after my walk and gratefully drank my SlimFast. For snack, I had an apple. I decided to take the boys to Taco Bell for lunch, where I had planned to have my usual bean burrito. Instead, I decided to try items off the Fresco menu. I had one crunchy taco and a chicken ranchero soft taco. They were good, and combined, less calories than my lone bean burrito. After I ate my lunch, I was miserably unsatisfied. I wanted two or three more tacos and had to wait patiently as my sons finished their lunches. A strange thing occurred when I got home – I realized I was full. Even though I was tempted at the restaurant, the food actually did its work and made me full. Full is a nice feeling. I took a brief rest (because the boys were loudly playing cards) and got up and had another apple. I wonder why? I usually take naps because of all the sugar I've been eating and typically crave something sweet upon waking. I had the same desire for something sweet right away and reached for the apple; I wonder if I should have ....

I needed to run some errands in Union City, so I took the boys to eat at Applebee's. I love eating there because of the Weight Watchers menu. I had the tilapia and a salad and some grapes in the car on the way home.

My Existential Eaters Society met tonight. What a great group of women! I know others have food issues, but it is comforting to hear of other's struggles and triumphs.

July 10, 2009
I went for a late walk, came home, and drank a SlimFast and later ate an apple for a snack. Today, we drove back to Kentucky to pick up my husband. I packed lunches for the trip and off we went. I had a peanut butter sandwich. I thought I'd be okay with the peanut butter because I wasn't eating it in the house. Even if I wanted more, I didn't have access to it. I ate my sandwich and looked at the clock ... I gave myself two hours to wait until I had my mid-day snack of V-8. I had the same problems I had on Monday – it is difficult to be in the car and not eat. I planned to stop at Subway on the way back home once we picked up Chris. The boys were too hungry to wait for the Subway exit, so we took an earlier exit and ended up at Denny's. Eating out on a Friday night is harder for me to find something healthy to eat because I try not to eat meat on Fridays. I ended up

eating breakfast: one pancake (no butter or syrup), 2/3 of a large yogurt, 2/5 of a bowl of oatmeal (no sugar), and a serving of fruit. The meal was yummy, though I worried I ate too much yogurt. As soon as I put the kids in bed, I got online to check the calories of the items I ate – mostly because I was still hungry and wanted to eat an apple. I know I'm on the extreme of obsessing over every-little-thing I put in my mouth. I'm a work in progress and hope I won't always be so uptight about food – better on my guard than beholden to my vicious appetites.

I weighed in this morning at 133.8. I lost a total of 6.2 pounds this month – not too shabby!

Appendix D: Binging and Purging while on the Last Diet Ever

Fast forward a few months to September of 2009.

Towards the end of my Last Diet Ever, I had a hard time keeping up my rigid food control. I had several binge eating episodes. I was in the middle of writing my unpublished diet book, and wrote about the experiences (see below), mostly to try to make sense of my behavior. While I was bothered by my actions I wasn't completely devastated because:

- I still retained the ability to not eat sugar.
- I was still writing down everything I ate, even if it was truly awful.
- I still awoke with the mindset of being on a diet.

While I could see the binges were due to the tyrannical control I had forced on my eating, I lacked the foresight and the tools to advert the disaster that was months away from taking me down.

The Binge

I obviously believe we are free to choose what we put into our bodies (those of us, at least, with access to money and food options). But how free are we? Our bodies need food; they must have food to survive. If we neglect to feed our bodies, our bodies fight back. What a balance to find! Don't eat too much or too little … but eat.

I believe I am solely responsible for what and how much I eat. I firmly believe this. So how do I explain my recent irrational binging behavior?

What is a binge? Eating too much at one meal? A second helping? No. This is a binge (and not just your average few hours binge, but a whole day affair):

1 SlimFast
3 cornbread pancakes
4 (or 5?) packages of peanut butter crackers (6 per pack)
8 to 9 cups of cheerios
4 packages of individually wrapped graham cracker treats (2 Scooby snacks and 2 bug bites)
3 bags of 100 calorie size popcorn
4 chicken patties (faux chicken – morning star)
2 diet cokes and 3 diet A&Ws
2 trips through the buffet line at Dragon Buffet

This is what I can recall of what I ate today, September 16, 2009 … there may have been more. This is more food than I've had in one day in over 16 months. This is usually about what I eat in one week! Why now? WHY EVER? Why would I treat my body with such carelessness, such wild abandon? Did I enjoy myself? Yes and no. I enjoyed the 'freedom' to eat whatever I wanted (without eating dessert – a non-option for me). Did I enjoy the food? Not really. I felt compelled to eat it.

I was sick. I was up late grading, Chris was asleep, and I knew the food was coming back up, or at least a part of it was. I really did not want the day to end that way. I needed to take responsibility for what I had eaten, which means I should deal with the belly ache and thousands of calories. My mind, however, was made up. I wanted to go to bed but felt too sick. I went to the bathroom and made myself throw up. Halfway through, I locked the door out of shame. How could I explain this to Chris when I could barely explain it to myself? As I stood over the toilet, I told myself I was only doing this because I was so sick to my stomach, and I was. But I couldn't help but wonder if I was being authentic about my motives.

I awoke the next morning with an unexpected smile. Different. I felt as if a burden was gone, a veil lifted. I've been wrapped up in knots for so long over what and what not to eat, when, and how much. I've been trying to exercise tight control on all things food, sometimes succeeding, usually falling a bit short and occasionally out-right failing in an extravagant manner.

I awoke understanding myself. I saw why I ate the way I did, the answer to the binge. I saw how my extreme anxiety over food and food choices had backed me into a corner, leading me to 'give myself permission' to binge whenever a crack in my will power showed. If I was allowing myself to eat something on my temporary 'no' list, why not anything and everything else I wanted? With my guard down I felt it was a one-time opportunity, for as soon as I could regain control those foods would be off limits again. Ever the child who does something devious because she can get away with it.

Did I enjoy what I ate on my binge? Not really. I would have been much happier going through McDonald's and getting a hamburger and fries – happier and I would have saved thousands of calories! It is interesting to me that I was able to function at such a high level while on this mammoth food binge.

I played with my baby a lot, pulled weeds, worked on the yard, hung out with my older boys after school, got a lot of grading done, and finished reading *Captain Underpants* to the older boys. And yet, with every move, I was either eating or planning what to consume next. How can one person eat almost an entire box of cereal, move on to the next item she can find, and still function? I did not yell at anyone and can't honestly say I was in a haze either. I knew what I was doing and did not want to stop … and, unfortunately, felt I could not stop. Why would I want to stop eating?

So, I ate. I was unsatisfied. With each bite I wanted more, never enough. Though I got tired of cereal and peanut butter crackers, I was not tired of eating. I will never tire of that activity. Never.

I saw this morning that food, for me, will never fill me. I am a bottomless pit when it comes to food. What difference does it make to shovel two tons of dirt into a bottomless pit … it has no bottom, no way *to be filled*, at least with dirt. Food will never fill me. I must give up on the fantasy, must let go, really let go, of this duplicitous lover.

So where does binging behavior lead me? Back to virtue of course. I now know a day and a half binge will not send me into eating healthy remission, where I fall off the wagon for years, whoring myself out to fast-food restaurants and any chocolate/dessert that comes my way. No. I am different.

This binging shows me, yet again, how very broken I am. There is much work to be done. On the outside I look 'fixed,' but as you know, this is a lie. My body now lies, is inauthentic, to those around me because I look 'fine.' Seeing *is not* believing. I am a mess, but I am happy to be looking at the mess I am – not looking away, running from my insanity.

I awoke with peace in my heart. This is yet another facet I have to deal with as I mend. What will help me gain control of my eating? The answer is in the question. Control will come about through continuing to work on having the virtues. All the virtues are my companions as I strive to be whole. Today, I saw the wisdom in mercy and patience. Mercy on my outrageous behavior and the patience to see I am in a process, a long, long, long (did I mention the process is long?) of healing.

Another binge

I thought I was through with this nonsense! This time I ate not as much as the time before, but enough to be sick. Sick enough to throw it all up. I am such an idiot! Do I really want to go down this losing path? This is not the path of wellness and recovery but of yet another unhealthy and deadly addiction. In my defense I was sick all day, with a temperature; I was not thinking clearly. If I'd had my wits about me, would it have even mattered?

When will this end? When will I make peace with food?

And thus, I see the value in the life of virtue. I see, for the first time in my life, that I am in a process. In order to be victorious, I must work on the virtues. I must call on patience to see me to the end. I must call on mercy, which I need to use daily to deal with my less than stellar eating performances. I must work to control my eating and eat in moderation.

Another binge, third purge, and the end of it

I moped around all day declaring to the walls how much I hate food. Done with food. I ate very well all day. Having eaten my veggie soup dinner when T (blame the baby!) wanted more food. This brought me to the kitchen and the realization that I hadn't eaten all my points for the day. So, I had 4 slices of low-calorie bread – a total of 160 calories, which actually was fine given what I'd eaten that day, and NOT fine for carbs have been doing me in as of late ... and then the dam broke. I ate peanut butter, popcorn, cups of cereal, three 100 calorie packs of cheese-it pack mixes, three packs of graham crackers, and one pack of Scooby-snack graham cracker packs as I walked to the uninhabited in-laws' house to throw it all up. What an absolute mess. And now, today, in the light of the sun it seems like another person did these stupid childish things. Not me, not an adult, married woman, mother of three, philosophy instructor.

And yet, this morning, the morning after, I knew this to be the last time. I will not purge again. If I do, I will make an appointment with a mental health professional and tell my husband ... the last is the scariest. He has been so understanding, patient, and tolerant with me. I know he won't (and I think shouldn't) tolerate this aberrant behavior.

On my walk this morning, I realized with whom I was fighting. The fight is not me vs. my body but me vs. my tongue. Is this really true? True to an extent. If so, why would I let such a little organ order me around? Why would I decide to listen to it over and against my pal reason?

The compulsion I've felt is so intensely strong, I've felt powerless to fight against it. Every ounce of my body flinches at the idea of binge eating being completely out of my control. This can't be the case. And even if it is partly true, I get to decide what to do in its aftermath. I decide to make a plan of action (or not) when I find myself starting to binge. I decide (or not) what to do after I've binged. A purge does not necessarily follow from binging. I decide.

I'm telling you my shameful behavior to give you hope. Is it hard to be controlled around food? Yes. Is it impossible to control yourself? No – not over the long haul. I look at this most recent disturbing behavior of mine as yet another hurdle as I charge ahead in the battle. I mess up and make a mess of things a lot, but I will not give up hope. Oh, my passions are greatly disappointed; they want to eat unfettered; they like it when I play the helpless fool. I want to be better than that. I want to be me, a human person, who chooses what her life is to be like.

The almost binge

My last binge/purge was on a Monday. The rest of the week went relatively smoothly. I felt in control, for the most part, of what I ate. Then came Saturday.

After a long walk, I had a SlimFast for breakfast. A few hours later, I had almost an entire bag of grapes. This should have been a warning to me, but I didn't see it ... it was just grapes, a yummy fruit that is good for the body. I headed out to the soccer field around 11:30 a.m. to see L's soccer game, which began at Noon. I debated as to whether to eat lunch before the game, during the game, or just wait until afterwards. I chose the latter because I wasn't really hungry yet (still full of the grapes!).

After the game, I had a very small window in which to get lunch for everyone, get J home and changed from soccer gear and into appropriate party gear for a birthday party that was already in progress. On the way home from the soccer field, we went through Taco Bell where I ordered a bean burrito. I ate it before we got home. Once home, I kicked everyone out of the car and got J dressed. As I was climbing back into the mini-van, I remembered the peanut butter crackers in the trunk – left over from this morning's games. What would it hurt if I had just one pack? I knew the possible damage, the possibility of opening the flood gates. Could I eat only one package? I ate one package and the fire began. I knew in my mind I needed nothing else to eat … yet I wanted, needed more. No.

"Today, I will not give in," I told myself repeatedly. I was able to see through the haze and an opportunity to begin to break the binging cycle. "Today, I will not binge," and it was going to cost me.

Once back from the non-party, (I got the day wrong!) I took a nap – avoidance. After the nap, the burning was waiting for me.

L and I decided to go to a 5 o'clock movie while the rest of my clan watched football. We saw a kid's movie all about food. Everyone around me was enjoying their treats, just as my son chewed his way through a pack of sour gummy worms. I drank my water.

I knew Chris, J, and T were having pizza for dinner. I told my husband on my way out the door the pizza was to be gone upon my return. Pizza and I are current enemies … I wish it weren't so. Home from the movies, I went to the kitchen to eat my vegetable soup. On the counter were two half eaten pizzas. I stared, I contemplated, I salivated like a dog. No.

Chris swooped into the kitchen, scooping all the leftovers into Tupperware and into the refrigerator. He moved so quickly, apologizing for not doing it sooner – like he got it. He understood how messed-up I am about food.

I ate my vegetable soup and a whole bag of frozen vegetables, read, and went to bed. A binge was avoided!

The next day

The next day comes, as always. Who knows what tomorrow holds for any one of us or what we will choose? I chose to binge. I had no intentions of doing so, of course, but I did. I was babysitting a bunch of kids at my friend's house. I already had a large lunch and apple afterwards. I could tell, even before I decided to binge, this day was going to be a struggle. At my friend's house, I had a peach and then I started eating. She had just come home from the store and had Naan bread. Delicious. I moved on to flour tortillas and ended my eating spree there with loads of pretzels.

After I returned home and dropped the kids off with Chris, I went to the grocery store where I got popcorn chicken to eat in the store. I then ended up in the aisle I was dreaming of – the cracker aisle. Must have graham crackers. I bought a 12 pack of individually packaged graham crackers and had consumed three before I left the store and another two on the way home. I was now sick.

Sick is a nice word for the way I felt. It was beautiful outside. Chris was barbequing chicken and playing with the boys outside. All I could do was go inside and lay on the bed – I had had it! What a mess I was. I went back outside and told Chris "I had a bad day" and his response was to hold me. He kissed my hair and encouraged me, telling me of my growth and that I am a person on the way, still working on my issues. What a lucky woman I am. I have a husband who loves me and tells me the truth.

I have decided to ban all forms of graham crackers for an entire year. Come end of September 2010, I will evaluate whether to admit them into my food cannon.

And then I went to lunch, where I ate the chips at La Canasta! I then went through the car to find the two packs of graham crackers I knew were there. I cannot relate to you adequately how very disappointing it is to not be able to trust yourself.

***

The rest of 2009 was a struggle where I binged occasionally, purged a few more times, all while finishing my diet book on finding freedom from food addiction through the virtues! The cracks had formed, though I had no idea what was in store for me.

At the beginning of 2010, I lost it. What I had been holding on to, through the binging and even the occasional purging, was the fact that I'd successfully given up dessert. So, when I ate the box of See's Candy, I was done. I had been psychologically defeated. This is when I went into months and months of binging. Not overeating. Binging. Binging in my car, in parking lots, in driveways that weren't mine, locked in the bathroom – crying while eating. Somehow, I decided it was a just punishment to not purge. I didn't purge out of a kind of self-inflected punishment.

I binged, ending my year and a half of restrictive eating. I gained all the weight back. My period returned (surprise, surprise). I developed BED and was thrown into a clinical depression.

Appendix E: Resources

Here are a few resources to aide you on your journey. For more online resources, links, and posts from what's going on in the culture visit me at merrybrownbooks.com.

The Twelve Steps of Overeaters Anonymous

1. We admitted we were powerless over food—that our lives had become unmanageable.
2. Came to believe that a Power greater than ourselves could restore us to sanity.
3. Made a decision to turn our will and our lives over to the care of God as we understood Him.
4. Made a searching and fearless moral inventory of ourselves.
5. Admitted to God, to ourselves and to another human being the exact nature of our wrongs.
6. Were entirely ready to have God remove all these defects of character.
7. Humbly asked Him to remove our shortcomings.
8. Made a list of all persons we had harmed, and became willing to make amends to them all.
9. Made direct amends to such people wherever possible, except when to do so would injure them or others.
10. Continued to take personal inventory and when we were wrong, promptly admitted it.
11. Sought through prayer and meditation to improve our conscious contact with God as we understood Him, praying only for knowledge of His will for us and the power to carry that out.

12. Having had a spiritual awakening as the result of these Steps, we tried to carry this message to compulsive overeaters and to practice these principles in all our affairs.

Overeaters Anonymous: https://oa.org/

National Eating Disorder Association:
https://www.nationaleatingdisorders.org/learn/by-eating-disorder/bed

Eating Disorder Hope: https://www.eatingdisorderhope.com/

National Association of Anorexia Nervosa and Associated Disorders: https://anad.org/

The Eating Disorder Foundation:
https://eatingdisorderfoundation.org/

US Department of Agriculture on eating disorders:
https://www.nutrition.gov/topics/diet-and-health-conditions/eating-disorders

www.ingramcontent.com/pod-product-compliance
Lightning Source LLC
Chambersburg PA
CBHW031431270326
41930CB00007B/652